Your Diet and Your Heart

by J. I. Rodale
and the Prevention staff

Rodale Books, Inc.
Emmaus, Penna. 18049

STANDARD BOOK NUMBER 87596-042-1

LIBRARY OF CONGRESS CATALOG CARD NUMBER 75-86523

COPYRIGHT 1969 BY J. I. RODALE

ALL RIGHTS RESERVED

PRINTED IN UNITED STATES

PB-27

FIRST PRINTING — JULY 1969

Contents

iii

iv

Introduction:

Can Heart Disease Be Prevented?

It will take 2,500,000,000 heartbeats to get you from the cradle to the grave—if your heart holds out. Chances that it won't are one in five, if you're a man between 45 and 60, or a woman over 65 years of age. Someone is killed by a heart attack every minute in this country. Many more—an estimated two million men and women—have had heart attacks and lived. Most of them, painfully aware that it could happen again, are living more carefully than they did before. And all of them wish they'd known as much about preventing the first heart attack as they've learned about preventing a second.

A significant preponderance of heart attacks could be anticipated and avoided if people would take the

[1]

trouble to analyze their own cardiac tendencies and take steps when they recognize danger signs.

Medical researchers have now put together a pretty good portrait of a heart attack about to happen. You should know if they're talking about you. If they are, now is the time to do something about it.

Menard M. Gertler, M.D., in his book *You Can Predict Your Heart Attack and Prevent It* (Random House), says the victim-to-be will have a square solid build with strong muscular features and firmly set jaw. He will be on the short side and have a thickish neck and wrists. He will be squat and probably look overweight, even if he is not. He might be anything from banker to truck driver; occupation doesn't matter. His father or mother or both have experienced heart attacks, and a brother or a sister may have had one too. If this same fellow mentions a few attacks of indigestion lately, or if he suffers from gout, diabetes, or high blood pressure, if he smokes and uses fair amounts of alcohol, he is pressing his luck if he hopes to get through life without a heart attack.

These are a few of the clues that add up to the "Coronary Profile." It is a listing of the factors involved in heart attack—those which can bring it on.

Statistics and experience have pretty well convinced doctors that a heart attack in the family will put you on the road to repeating the same experience. There are more fathers and mothers of coronary patients who have themselves experienced heart attacks than there are patients' parents who have not. And if you have a heart attack, there are eight times as many chances that

[2]

your brother or sister will have had one too than that the brother or sister of a healthy person will have had heart trouble.

Your Body Type

Your body shape helps to determine how likely you are to have a heart attack. Stand nude in front of a mirror and you will see that you fall into one of three body types. You will be predominantly soft and round, or muscular and angular in outline, or long boned and fragile, with tapering fingers and toes. W. H. Sheldon, M.D., in a study of 97 heart attack patients at Massachusetts General Hospital, showed that the rounded and fat-prone body build, and the muscular, angular persons are the most likely candidates for a heart attack.

Few people who are too fat need charts and listings to tell them so. What is important is to face it and to know that it's dangerous. Look at yourself unclothed in the mirror and pinch up your skin in several places. The skin fold you pinch is mostly pure fat. Every pound of flab brings you closer to heart attack. Even if you weigh the same, a great deal of what was muscle in your college days may be fat now. Your eyes are often better judges than a scale.

Cholesterol's Role

Excessive intake of animal fat, sugar or both is believed to be the major cause of a high cholesterol level, generally considered a danger to heart health. If your cholesterol count is high, researchers urge a limit to the quantity of sweets and of fatty meats, butter, cheese,

[3]

UYIC ACID

milk, etc. which contain the cholesterol-rich fats that
are solid at room temperature. Vegetable oils, in their
liquid non-hydrogenated form, (corn oil, olive oil, soy
oil, etc.) contain important elements (linoleic acid, for
one) which help the body to process the hydrogenated
fats it does take in, and to use cholesterol so that it
does not form plaques which can plug up an artery to
slow the flow of blood and make the heart work harder.
When vegetable oils are processed or even when they
are used for frying at home, they become oxidized to
rancidity and present just as much of a peril to the
body as the animal fats.

Gout, a painful, disabling relative to heart disease,
occurs with an overload of metabolic wastes which
show up in the blood as uric acid. It, too, is predominantly a male disease, and there is also a hereditary
predisposition to gout. The coronary arteries are more
likely to be prematurely diseased when gout is in the
picture. For these reasons gout and high uric acid readings are considered danger signs in predicting a heart
attack.

Associated Diseases

High blood pressure, which means that the heart
must work harder to push the blood through narrowed
arteries, strongly indicates the presence of a heart
problem. If this extra pressure is continued, the heart
muscle must eventually enlarge to carry out the extra
work load. With enlargement, the coronary arteries
must carry more blood which will increase pressure
within the arteries and lead to a narrowing of the

[4]

arterial channel. This narrower artery carrying more blood than it can handle will spell disaster if not relieved.

Diabetics are unable to handle sugars and starches. The metabolism disturbance spreads to the use of fats and proteins, and the small arteries of kidneys, eyes, legs, and heart are affected. Diabetes, even if controlled, speeds the physiological aging of the individual, particularly hardening of the arteries.

Does tobacco influence the incidence of heart disease? Most experts say it does. It makes the heart work faster and narrows the arteries. There are more smokers in a coronary group than in a non-coronary group. Among those who smoke, the coronary patients are the heavier smokers. The association between smoking and heart disease is very strong, and the smoker should take these findings into consideration.

Unfair as it may seem, just being a male will cause you to lose points on the coronary profile. From birth, the infant boy's blood vessels have a much thicker internal lining, consequently a smaller opening than the girl's. Arteriosclerosis and high blood pressure have a head start. Up to the age of forty, twenty-four men will experience heart attacks for every woman who does.

It is considered significant that heart attacks in women increase at the age of menopause, when a woman stops producing the female hormone, estrogen. Evidence that estrogen might be a protection for the heart shows up in women who have had their ovaries removed surgically early in life. They have more heart attacks than women of the same age group whose

[5]

ovaries are intact. Doctors say they can reinforce the female resistance to heart attack after menopause by giving compensating dosages of estrogen. Women treated in this way are relatively free and immune to coronary heart disease, but the hormone's side effects create other serious problems.

Just as the female hormone estrogen is believed to play a part in preventing heart disease in women, the male hormone testosterone might be responsible for male susceptibility to it. One large group of males, aged 18 to 80, whose organs for producing testosterone were removed for medical reasons, showed not a single sign of coronary artery disease. Even in postmortem examinations there was not a trace of this trouble.

If you are a man with a history of heart attacks whose level of blood serum cholesterol is high and who exhibits a prohibitive uric acid reading, you must consider the probability of heart attack as a real one. Are you overweight, is your body build one of the two riskier types, do you eat a diet high in animal fats, do you smoke and drink? If you have the wrong answers to the majority of these questions, you could be on the verge of serious trouble.

Alton Blakeslee and Jeremiah Stamler, M.D., in their book, *Your Heart Has Nine Lives* (Prentice-Hall), go to great lengths to prove that even a high risk individual needn't be counted out, and reasonable care can give him every chance of living a normal life span. "Your heart is the sturdiest, toughest muscle of your body. It is designed to beat steadily day and night without complaint for a century or longer." The important

[6]

thing is to clear away as many obstacles to its good health as possible.

Blakeslee and Stamler concentrate heavily on cholesterol and on ways to fight its increase in your blood. They offer an ideal anticholesterol menu. It includes fish, poultry, lean meats, baked or broiled (served without gravy or sauce), salads, plain vegetables, gelatin and fruits. The diet suggested here is a far cry from the regular fried food, high fat, high carbohydrate, high sweet diet that most Americans gobble every day.

Lose Weight Now

This diet not only raises cholesterol levels, but it also piles on extra pounds. At middle age the overweight man is two to three times more susceptible to coronary disease than his neighbor of normal weight. The answer to overweight is not "going on a diet," but eating more sensibly.

Nothing succeeds in a magazine or a book like a weight reducing diet. Americans love them. They will latch on to a 900 calorie diet, or a strict liquid diet, or a diet that allows only black coffee and rice, with a zest that is astounding. They even lose weight, but as the enthusiasm wears off the weight goes back on. Severe swings in weight loss and gain are harmful to your body.

Nine Lives offers a lot of good suggestions on how to get rid of the calories that you already have. The idea is to spend calories generously through exercise as an aid in fighting excess pounds. But whether you exercise

[7]

to lose weight or just for the fun of it, there are few things that you could do that would be of more benefit to your heart. Exercise or hard physical work makes the heart work harder and more efficiently. It develops what is known as collateral circulation—that is, a richer, more extensive network of blood channels to bring an even better blood supply to all areas of the heart muscle. And it helps to normalize cholesterol levels.

Books such as *You Can Predict Your Heart Attack and Prevent It* and *Your Heart Has Nine Lives* can make you so scared of heart failure that you will waste your life, afraid of overdoing, convinced that disaster or death waits around the corner; or they can lead you to a positive attitude about your health, one that will make you do what you must to prevent the disaster of a heart attack. The first step in the latter, constructive viewpoint is a good medical checkup, if you feel that you are in danger of heart trouble.

A heart attack does not have to be the end of everything. Many who are stricken in this way learn to live with the problem and to continue a useful life, giving beneficial service. Former Presidents Eisenhower and Johnson are two prime examples of recovery from severe heart attacks. But to invite heart attack through careless living, no matter what your chances of full recovery might be, is foolish and stupid. You must avoid the first heart attack before it happens.

It should be possible.

Europe is doing much better than we are at preventing heart disease. The Russian incidence of heart disease is the lowest in any civilized country in the world, and ours is the highest. The reason is simple enough: they concentrate on preventing heart trouble and we put all of our energy into treating it after it occurs. But we all know that the prevention of disease saves more lives, and it's easier on everybody. It's a scandal that American medicine has advanced so little in the field of preventive medicine.

It can't be that our doctors don't know how to go about organizing a preventive medicine program. There are blueprints for just what to do available from countries all over the world. In the *New Physician* (May, 1964) W. Raab, M.D., of the University of Vermont, President of the Preventive Heart Reconditioning Foundation, describes the program being used in the Soviet Union and other communist countries. The governments of these countries have constructed nearly three thousand rural reconditioning centers, where about 5 million fatigued and tense workers are admitted every year for four weeks of environmental, emotional relaxation and systematic physical training. While they are there, the people are taught rules for good health, proper exercise and proper diet which are intended to stay with them for a lifetime. These measures are continued daily, on a lesser scale, in the factories where there are regular exercise breaks and radio-conducted morning calisthenics for everyone. The idea is to re-establish the proper balance of the nervous system and, in turn, the health of the heart, which can be undermined by the over-civilized, sedentary, highly industrialized societies in which we live.

[9]

Centers in the Alps

In West Germany, Switzerland and Austria, private industry and insurance companies conduct similar programs. There are reconditioning centers in the Alps and the Black Forest which are expected to make a big difference in the cardiac death rate among the people of these countries. Already among the workers who have been trained in these centers, the absentee figures have dropped nearly 70 per cent within two years.

American Public Health authorities have made some feeble indication that they are interested in the results being achieved in Europe. In 1963 thirteen representatives of the American Public Health and Preventive Medicine Departments visited some of the West German reconditioning centers at the invitation of the German government. It was expected that the trip would result in steps toward the organization of preventive measures in the United States. However, at this time, there is still no plan for positive action in the work.

We Can Start Simply

It is reasonable to realize that a great deal of money, planning and personnel would be necessary to do the job here that is being done in Europe. But we could make a worthwhile and uncomplicated start by educating our people to the needless hazards to heart health they are subjected to every day. Many people don't realize, until they get to the doctor's office (if then), that the extra weight they carry might be

[10]

enough to turn them into heart disease victims. They never hear about the need for some exercise to keep the heart functioning properly and healthily. When they think about exercise, they think of it only in terms of calisthenics and weightlifting. No one ever tells them that a regular walk can do wonders for the heart, or that the frequent use of stairs in the homes can give them the exercise they miss by riding in a car and using an elevator. No one ever tells them that supplementary vitamin E can help to prevent stroke by limiting the chances of blood clot and enhancing the efficiency of the work the heart does.

Why don't doctors talk more about diet in relation to a healthy heart? Every doctor knows that salt is a strong factor in the development of high blood pressure. But the man on the street never hears about the problems salt can cause until he is in a doctor's office flushed and worried about a blood pressure that is in the stratosphere. Patients pop anti-cholesterol pills into their mouths at an enormous rate, only to find out later that the pills are dangerous and must be withdrawn from the market at the FDA's insistence. Researchers know that nicotinic acid, a B vitamin, is an effective anti-cholesterol agent. Choline and pyridoxine, two other B vitamins, have also been mentioned as valuable agents in reducing cholesterol accumulations in the blood. Lecithin is abundant in egg yolks and extremely important in cutting excess cholesterol in the blood stream. But whoever hears any strong publicity urging healthy people to eat B-rich foods and eggs to avoid heart disease? Only recently Dr. John Yudkin proved

[11]

a direct relationship between the amount of refined sugar we eat and the incidence of heart disease.

These factors illustrate the value of a good diet, rich in nutrients and natural foods, in maintaining the health of the heart. Modern American medicine gives the impression that Americans need be little concerned about adjusting their diet. Doctors say it automatically, without considering the loss in food values processing favorite American foods costs.

It is easy to see that much can be done in the field of heart disease prevention, whether we go all the way as the Europeans have done, or whether we limit ourselves to creating a greater awareness of the hazards to heart health involved in modern living. But surely we must start somewhere, we must do something. Our people need help in keeping their health, and they are looking to the government and organized medicine to provide it.

Part One:

YOUR HEART AND VITAMIN E

CHAPTER I

Conserving Oxygen in the Blood

Half of all American men over age 40 are statistically scheduled for a heart attack brought on by coronary atherosclerosis. This hardening of the coronary artery comes on gradually, and steadily decreases the blood supply to the heart muscle. The lack of oxygen that results causes dizziness or severe chest pain (angina pectoris), or both.

To detect hardening of the coronary artery, a doctor must rely largely on the patient's experiences. (If he tires easily and chest pain or dizziness comes with exertion, these are strong clues.) Objective diagnosis is difficult because the heart rate seems normal at rest, no abnormality is evident in the size or the shape of the heart and difficulties don't show up in electrocardiograms. Even the degree of pain is no true indication; it may range from mild to severe, and may appear in the arms, neck or jaws, as well as the chest. But when severe chest pain, brought on by effort, lasts longer than 15 or 20 minutes most doctors assume coronary thrombosis and treat it as such until other evidence is presented.

The classical treatments for angina pectoris are nitroglycerine tablets, or other nitrite compounds, and decreased activity. The nitroglycerine and nitrite compounds dilate the coronary artery, and relieve the pain, but the effect doesn't last and the drugs don't attack the cause of the problem. Alpha tocopherol (vitamin E) can actually conserve needed oxygen and this should make it the drug of choice in such cases.

In their book, *Alpha Tocopherol in Cardiovascular Disease*, Doctors W. E. Shute and E. V. Shute state that in full therapeutic doses—300 to 600 international units per day—vitamin E apparently reduces the oxygen requirement of the heart muscle. It accomplishes this in varying degree and at different dosage levels in different patients. Most patients with moderate or mild degrees of coronary insufficiency find their oxygen requirements reduced to a point at which activity, no matter how strenuous, will not cause pain. "Some with very marked degrees of coronary insufficiency, with angina pectoris elicited by even mild exertion or excitement, nevertheless lose all symptoms on alpha tocopherol therapy, because of a correspondingly great reduction in oxygen requirement."

This is not to say that every patient on alpha tocopherol can handle every kind of exertion, but the exercise tolerance is returned toward normal at varying

[16]

degrees. About eight out of ten of the patients who take alpha tocopherol for angina pectoris are definitely improved. Not merely relieved from pain, but improved.

The Shutes insist that every patient with angina pectoris should receive a full therapeutic dose of alpha tocopherol, if only because of its power as an anti-coagulant. According to K. L. Zierler, M.D., writing in the *American Journal of Physiology* (153:127, 1948), vitamin E is probably a major anti-coagulant in the human blood stream and when it is present in normal concentrations blood clots simply do not occur. When a patient suffers from angina pectoris, alpha tocopherol greatly increases his chances of avoiding a thrombosis, whether it improves his tolerance for exertion or not.

Finally, alpha tocopherol is known to prevent or relieve arterial contractions. It may also halt or even reverse the clogging changes that occur in the blood vessel walls.

Vitamin E is the only drug available which has any effect upon the basic causes of angina pectoris. No other drug can claim to halt or reverse the course of this painful and frightening disease.

Middle-aged men are most susceptible to angina, but it can happen to anyone—women included. Each of us must strive to maintain the highest natural concentration of oxygen in our blood streams. Vitamin E is the best means we have of doing this, so we should be concerned about getting our necessary quota every day. Supplementary vitamin E is a protective device we all can use to maintain a healthy circulatory system.

[17]

CHAPTER II

A Cure for Heart Disease

Wilfrid E. Shute, M.D.
Chief Cardiologist, Shute Institute for Clinical and
Laboratory Medicine, London, Ontario
(Reprinted from the *Vitamin E Bulletin*)

Most Important Discovery in Century

Actually, this heading is perhaps no exaggeration, much as one blushes to say it. It bids fair to be the most important discovery made in medicine in the last 100 years! Not excepting penicillin. This is due to two factors. The first concerns the appearance of a disease, new since 1900, called coronary thrombosis, characterized by the appearance of a clot in the coronary artery shutting off the blood supply to a segment of heart muscle. If instant death does not occur, as it may in one-quarter to one-third of those attacked, then the majority of such patients are seriously and critically ill for several weeks, and never return to normal health. Some are able to carry on their former occupations, some live a restricted life, and some are made permanent invalids. The disease has a characteristic tendency to recur, and fresh attacks add further damage to an already obviously damaged organ. The man who recovers merely waits for his next attack, and until recently medicine could not tell him how to ward it off.

Disease First Described in 1912

This disease was first described in 1912. It did not occur at autopsy in 1900, yet in 1951 it killed half the males who died over the age of 40. Included have been many famous and titled men; executives are particularly prone to this disease and it seems to have a peculiar selectivity for doctors.

The disease is increasing steadily, the number of deaths in 1951 showing an appreciable increase over the deaths in 1950, actually by 2 per cent in the U.S.A. In the last years for which we have data, 1949 and 1950, cardiovascular disease increased 9 per cent in Canada. In the last 10 years deaths from heart disease have increased by 45 per cent in Canada. We should stress this point which is never mentioned. This disease will almost certainly be much more deadly 10 years hence than it is now—perhaps by nearly 50 per cent. Isn't that a dreadful thought?

At first the disease chiefly affected older men of 60 years or more, but as it became more common it attacked more and more of the younger men until now

[19]

it is found in the late "teens," is not too rare in the 20's, and is rampant among the 30's and 40's.

Greatest Death Cause in World Today

It is the greatest single cause of death in the world today! It is becoming the way to die. It kills more people annually than all the atom bombs that any foreign nation could drop on this continent. While we shiver before the atom bomb, this one is falling on us steadily. In 1950—518,569 died in the U.S.A. and 38,718 died in Canada.

The second reason for the importance of this therapeutic suggestion of ours bears upon a peculiar function of vitamins, characteristic of all vitamins, namely, that they tend to prevent whatever disease or diseases they relieve and so this therapy opens up the way not only for the treatment of this, our own generation, who are already doomed to the encroachment of this dread disease, but it holds out hope of prevention for the generation of our children and grandchildren. That the most dreadful single disease confronting mankind today, not tuberculosis, not cancer, but coronary heart disease, can be completely wiped out within the next 50 years is the major and most hopeful implication of our treatment of coronary heart disease by Vitamin E.

Depends on Four Characteristics

The power of Vitamin E to treat and prevent heart disease of all types, whether coronary or rheumatic, depends upon four chief characteristics:

[20]

(1) Vitamin E seems to be a natural anti-thrombin in the human blood stream. It has been found by Zierler of Johns Hopkins and the U.S. Navy Research Department and Kay at Tulane to be a substance normally circulating in the blood of all men which prevents clots occurring inside the vessel. It is the only substance preventing the clotting of blood which is not dangerous. It does not interfere with the normal clotting of blood in a wound or with the normal healing process. Indeed it actually accelerates the healing of burns and wounds.

(2) The second important effect of the use of Vitamin E is oxygen conservation. It is a natural antioxidant in the body. It has been shown by Houchin and Mattill, and this has been confirmed by many workers, to decrease the oxygen requirement of muscle by as much as 43 per cent, and makes the narrow stream of blood which gets through the narrowed coronary artery in many heart patients adequate to prevent the occurrence of anoxia (lack of oxygen), which is the trigger that sets off angina or heart pain. Consequently, we have patients in Montreal who were once unable to walk half a block without the occurrence of angina pectoris but are now able to climb Mount Royal. Indeed, there is present in my audience today at least one such patient.

(3) The third major function of Vitamin E is the prevention of excessive scar tissue production and even, in some instances, the ability to melt away unwanted scar. It has been proven to function in this way in many areas of the body—from the hand, in Dupuytren's

[21]

contraction (Rochester, N.Y.)—to urinary tract strictures (Johns Hopkins).

(4) It is a dilator of blood vessels. This was beautifully demonstrated by X-ray in rabbits injected before and after the administration of Vitamin E by two workers in Florence, Italy. It opens up new pathways in the damaged circulation, therefore, and bypasses blocks produced by clot and hardened arteries.

Four Functions Extensively Confirmed

These four functions, all of them extensively confirmed in animal experimentation and human clinical work, make it the most valuable ally the cardiologist has yet found in the treatment of heart disease. It has no rivals. No other substance has this array of needful properties. This drug then becomes the first safe drug which can be given to patients suffering from the results of a clot in a coronary artery. There has been and still is no treatment at all for this type of case except two mildly useful drugs, which can be administered with great peril to the already precarious patient. Vitamin E replaces "rest and reassurance," which have no authentic basis, with real help to the damaged, laboring heart itself. It is the key to both the prevention and treatment of all those conditions in which a lack of blood supply due to thickened or blocked blood vessels or a lack of oxygen is a major or the whole story of the disease. As I have said, it has no rivals. No pharmacologist or internist can suggest another substance with all the powers and properties of this vitamin. God made it unique and we ignore it at our peril.

[22]

Work Declared World Famous

This work is world famous. Some 96 medical papers, not including our own, have already been written in its support. How many does one need to win his case?

Our work seems to have been the source of Ochsner's studies on the prevention of post-operative clotting by the use of Vitamin E, of the work of many Italian workers on heart disease, of Professor Boyd's (of the University of Manchester) published treatment of intermittent claudication (Buerger's disease to you) and with phlebitis; of much recent work on diabetes mellitus. Indeed, the treatment of diabetes mellitus nowadays requires three agents, not two; these are: a balanced diet, insulin and Vitamin E! Any one or two alone are not adequate. The three form a nearly unbeatable combination. Everyone interested in treating diabetes now is aware of the deplorable results achieved by the use of insulin and diet only.

160 Medical Men Patients in Institute

We have over 160 medical men as personal patients at our institute. We know of many more who are taking it on their own. Presumably what is good enough for them is good enough for their patients. Early this month one appeared who had been a successful surgeon in California. After a heart attack he had been given Vitamin E by his doctor. He merely came to us for regulation of his dosage. He used these words to me: "Everybody is using it for treatment of heart disease in California!"—a pleasant but slight exaggeration, perhaps.

[23]

There is much animal experimentation to show that this drug may be the key to the control of hardening of the arteries. I cannot help but recall the words of the great pathologist, Gideon Wells, under whom I studied pathology for 15 months, who told me that the man who discovered the prevention and treatment of arteriosclerosis had found the key to eternal youth. A man is as old or as young as his arteries.

I would, if I had time, give you in detail the results of some of these experiments. I could tell you of the work of Tusini in Italy, who showed that a substance like Ergotamine tartrate which caused spasm of the arteries in rats could be neutralized by Vitamin E, and that giving Vitamin E to the animal ahead of time would protect him against the action of this drug. I would like to tell you about the workers who showed that deposition of cholesterol in the wall of the arteries in rabbits force-fed cholesterol could be prevented by Vitamin E.

Can Be Added to "Wonder" Drug List

We think that Vitamin E can safely be added to the list of so-called "wonder" drugs. No one knows precisely the mode of action of any of these, but that they act and on what they act are matters of common knowledge. It was not always so. It took 14 years from the first investigation of penicillin before it came into general use, but the doctor who was responsible for this is now Lady Florey.

We are happy to have been instrumental in discovering the use of Vitamin E in treating cardiovascular

[24]

disease, not only coronary thrombosis, but rheumatic and hypertensive heart disease where it is also very effective; in discovering the value of Vitamin E in many diseases of the arteries in the extremities. We are proud of the considerable number of legs which should by this time be in pathological museums, but are still serving their owners in everyday life, climbing roofs, dancing, playing pipe-organs, even soldiering.

We, of course, hope to continue our work. Our institute has more opportunity for worth-while cardiovascular research work than any medical institution in Canada has now or has ever had. It is our constant regret that our days are filled with nothing but seeing the sick, important and merciful as that is, but we realize that this will not always be so. In the past year, we have had to turn down requests from Spanish, Indian, Syrian and German research men to join our staff since we have neither the time nor facilities for their work here.

Over 8,600 Patients Treated

We have now personally treated over 8,600 cardiovascular patients. My great regret is that circumstances today prevent me showing you some of our hundreds of colored photographs of these people. I wonder how many people realize that this is many times the number seen in a comparable time elsewhere. We are no longer reporting on our first 10 cases. We are reporting to you on the conclusions derived from thousands. It is an investigation that Canadians and Canada should be proud of, for in this at least they lead the world.

[25]

CHAPTER III

The Record of Vitamin E

In the *American Journal of Physiology,* volume 153, page 127, 1948, K. L. Zierler, D. Grob and J. L. Lilienthal describe laboratory experiments in which they discovered that vitamin E has a profound effect on the blood, especially the clotting of the blood. It has a strong anti-clotting effect both in laboratory experiments and in the veins and arteries of human beings. Now there is a special natural substance in the blood called heparin which is made in the liver, whose job it is to prevent the coagulation of blood. In their tests these scientists found that the action of vitamin E on the blood takes place regardless of how much or how little heparin is present in the blood stream of the patients. So there can be no doubt but that the anticoagulating action is the result of the vitamin E and nothing else.

In an Italian journal, *Bollettino Societa Chirurgia,* volume 18, page 155 (1948), R. Castagna and G. Impallomeni report on seven patients with phlebitis (inflammation of a vein) and one 71-year-old woman who had an ulcer measuring five by three inches on her lower leg. The phlebitis responded dramatically to the use of vitamin E alone. The woman patient's ulcer healed in 26 days. The authors have also used vitamin E in treatment of vascular disease (any disease of the blood vessels) and for "strokes." They tell us that in thrombophlebitis (inflammation of the vein in which a blood clot is involved) the improvement by using vitamin E is extremely rapid. In addition, they say, treatment with vitamin E does not require rigid blood control as do other medications.

From Brazil (Publication of the O Hospital for July 1949) D. de Olivera describes two cases of phlebitis, one during a pregnancy and one following childbirth. In both cases fever fell rapidly and there was no recurrence of the disease when the first patient had her child. The conservative British medical publication, *The Lancet,* volume 2, page 132, 1949, carries an article by A. M. Boyd, A. H. James, G. W. H. and R. P. Jepson saying that clinical results with vitamin E are far better than any obtained with any other treatment in cases of obliterative diseases of the blood vessels. It can be used most successfully for the relief of cramps in the calves of the legs. "May we repeat," say these authors, "that it is our considered opinion that the clinical observations so far made warrant the continued use of vitamin E therapy."

[27]

O. Mantero, B. Rindi and L. Trozzi, writing in the Italian magazine *Attivita Congresso degli Cardiologia,* Stresa, May 1948, discuss five cases of acute and subacute phlebitis which were rapidly healed by vitamin E therapy. J. H. Kay, S. B. Weiss, G. H. and A. Ochsner mention in *Surgery,* volume 28, page 124, 1950, four cases of phlebitis treated only with vitamin E given orally in which "inflammation subsided and the swelling disappeared."

A Norwegian physician, H. Sturup, writing in *Nordisk Medicin,* volume 43, page 721, 1950, tells us he has seen a number of cases of thrombosis helped by vitamin E therapy. He discusses in detail the case of a 33-year-old patient who had chronic phlebitis of the left leg, five years after an operation. This patient was not even confined to bed, but took vitamin E daily and within six days the pain and swelling disappeared.

The *Annals of Surgery,* volume 131, page 652, 1950, reports that vitamin E and calcium appear to be helpful in the treatment of vascular diseases. Dr. A. W. Allen of Boston, commenting on this article, tells us that he has used vitamin E on a number of patients and can report that 50 of these who were "vulnerable" —that is susceptible—to thrombosis escaped this serious condition. This seems to us particularly important, for in these cases vitamin E was used to prevent rather than to cure, and fifty lucky patients continued in good health. Dr. J. C. Owings of Baltimore comments that he has treated many leg ulcers due to phlebitis with a combination of rutin and vitamin E, all of which stayed

[28]

healed, so long as the patient continued to take the medication.

Postgraduate Medicine, volume 10, page 794, 1951, carries a report by A. Ochsner who believes that vitamin E is the best preventive of a blood clot, because it is a natural substance, so there is no hazard involved in its use. The use of other anticoagulants is dangerous and tying off veins should not be practiced because it will not protect against the detachment of clots. He states that he does not know whether vitamin E combined with calcium is the final answer, but adds that it seems to be best, because it is perfectly safe and does not bring any danger of producing bleeding.

Medical Thesis, published in Paris, Number 471, 1951, quotes a physician as saying he has found vitamin E and calcium useful for preventing blood clots after surgery. R. Bauer, writing in *Wiene Klinische Wochenschrift,* a German publication, volume 31, page 552, 1951, says Dr. Ochsner's method can be used successfully in reducing one-tenth of the usual incidence of thrombosis and should perhaps be used to decrease the danger of clot in coronary thrombosis. M. Reifferscheid and P. Matis, writing in *Medizinische Welt,* Germany, volume 20, page 1168, 1951, announce they have found vitamin E to be definitely protective against vascular clotting. They found that large daily doses were necessary. They describe five cases of diabetic gangrene, nine cases of Raynaud's disease (a gangrenous condition), seven cases of Dupuytren's contracture (contraction of tissues under the skin of the palm) and

[29]

14 cases of hemorrhagic (bleeding) diseases which all yielded to treatment with vitamin E.

Dr. W. E. Crump and E. F. Heiskell, writing in the *Texas State Journal of Medicine,* volume 11, 1952, agree that the use of the regular anti-coagulants for routine prevention of clotting diseases in patients after operations is too dangerous for general use. In most cases where these medicines are used, as many patients die of hemorrhage as might have died of clots and 16 per cent of other cases develop non-fatal bleeding complications. When vitamin E was used as treatment by these physicians no bleeding occurred and only minor side reactions were noticed. When cases of phlebitis occurred during treatment, they were mild and had no complications. There were no lung clots, fatal or non-fatal, in patients being treated with vitamin E. Dr. Terrell Speed, commenting on these statements, says "considerable evidence is accumulating to substantiate the value of this therapy. However I have gradually expanded its use and now it is used routinely in essentially the same group of cases mentioned by the authors. If the promising preliminary results are borne out, relative protection against one of the most feared complications of surgery will have been obtained."

Two German physicians, S. Schmid writing in *Wiene Klinische Wochenschrift,* volume 64 and H. Wagner writing in *Aerztliche Wochenschrift,* volume 7, page 248, 1952, say they have achieved good results in treating thrombosis with vitamin E.

If you have no difficulty with your heart or circula-

[30]

tion, we suggest that you take vitamin E and/or wheat germ oil so that you will at all times have an abundance of vitamin E and will run no risk of suffering a deficiency. A minimum daily requirement of vitamin E has not been set in this country, so no one can tell you officially how much you should take every day. Follow the dosage recommended on the bottle in which your wheat germ oil or vitamin E comes to you. Considering that heart patients in a weakened condition take enormous doses of pure vitamin E, there is little chance that you can get too much. And if you habitually eat products made from white flour from which the germ has been removed, if your diet is short on vegetable oils and green leafy vegetables, there's every reason to believe that you are not now getting enough vitamin E for full protection.

A Prevention *Reader Gives Her Experiences With Vitamin E*

Here is a completely unsolicited letter from a *Prevention* reader who did just what we suggested above, when she discovered that she was beginning to have trouble with her heart. Please note that this is not a miraculous, overnight cure. Mrs. Paetz is still taking vitamin E and will for perhaps a long time to come. But note, too, the wonderful change from despair to hope, note the improvement, the confidence, the well being.

"Dear Mr. Rodale:

"I had always thought I was pretty healthy because the only times I had ever the occasion to see a doctor

[31]

was for physicals for positions I held, my pre-marital examination and my pre- and post-natal care when I carried my one and only baby, now a doll of eight years.

"Then about two years ago I began having some pretty gruesome symptoms: chest pains, extreme heaviness in the chest, difficulty in taking a deep breath, extreme weakness and undefined fear, such as I'd never known. I was so afraid—of what I don't know—that I would not go twenty feet from my door unless my mother (who lives on the first floor) or some member of my family went with me. All this from a gal who used to take her baby miles from home both in the baby carriage and in a bus or taxi!

"At first, although I was very ill, I procrastinated— didn't want my husband to know how really bad I felt, and passed most of it off as 'nerves.' I took Nervine by the bottleful and of course, since it deadened some of my senses, I did get a little relief. Then when that didn't work any more, I attributed my aches, pains, feelings of pressure and suffocation, etc., to fifteen pounds I had put on since marriage. But the day came when I couldn't procrastinate any longer. I went to a doctor who had been highly recommended. After hearing all my symptoms, he immediately put me under the fluoroscope. Fortunately for me he found my lungs and heart of normal size and seemingly normal in their functions. But, when he examined my heart under the stethoscope, his very expression changed and he asked 'Did you ever know that you have a very loud heart murmur? It's probably something you carried over from childhood.' A loud heart murmur! And it

[32]

accounted for my awful symptoms. Then I remembered my mother telling me that my brothers and I had had only one childhood disease, but it was a bad one— scarlet fever! (And just a year ago my little girl had scarlet fever too.) When I told the doctor what my mother had told me, he said, 'I'm sure your heart was damaged then, but now you'll just have to live with it. I'm going to give you some medication and some medicine to help you take off 15 pounds.'

"When I got home I took the mail from the mail box and one of the items was the August *Prevention*. Imagine my delight when I read the article titled 'Vitamin E, Cure for Heart Disease.' It wasn't till October of 1952 that I contacted Dr. Wilfrid E. Shute and on October 15, 1952 under his personal supervision began taking 90 milligrams of vitamin E daily, to be increased to 120 milligrams daily and later up to 300 milligrams. Of course, I had to be certain that my E came from entirely natural and not synthetic sources. During these first early weeks there were no dramatic results — but there certainly were about Thanksgiving. With extra guests, stress and strain, lots more work (especially for one in my condition) I should have been feeling it, as it were. Instead I was actually feeling swell! I was breathing normally and not gasping every time I did more than walk straight! I suddenly realized that I didn't have that terrible heavy feeling on my chest and that those vague aches and pains in my chest were gone. My heart had quieted down to the point where I was no longer conscious of my own heart beats, flutters and palpitations, simply

[33]

because my heart was beating normally and I no longer had those other abnormal sensations. This I definitely attribute to taking vitamin E on Dr. Wilfrid E. Shute's advice.

"Also after having *Prevention* as a welcome guest in my home for over a year now, I realize the truths of the statements that our so-called 'wholesome good food' is not what it's cracked up to be, but filled with poisons and so forth to keep the color good, to improve the keeping qualities and to enrich those things that have been tampered with and contaminated in the first place. As a result, I bought wheat germ, wheat germ oil capsules, natural sea kelp for iodine, vitamin A and D capsules, fresh garlic and garlic perles, desiccated liver tablets and, because our water is heavily chlorinated, I now buy mineral water by the case. Of course it's expensive, but it all enabled me to throw the doctor's prescription down the drain and for me, it enabled me to regain a semblance of my former self, with vigor and vitality in spite of a 'heart' ailment. My little girl, too, has enjoyed a year of perfect health because of the natural food supplements, and, God willing, we'll go on this way."

Early Vitamin E Successes

In view of the overwhelming evidence that vitamin E is a most valuable aid that should long ago have been harnessed by the medical profession, it is difficult to understand why this has not been done. The puzzling attitude of the medical profession, with regard to vitamin E, caused *Macleans* magazine of Canada to make

[34]

its own investigation. *Macleans* is considered the *Saturday Evening Post* of Canada. It is a long-established, conservative and widely-read magazine of large circulation. It assigned one of their best men, Eric Hutton, to do a thorough investigation and journalistic job, and his article on the subject was printed in the June 15, 1953 issue of the magazine.

Eric Hutton has done painstaking research among friends and enemies of vitamin E therapy for heart disease, has talked to physicians, members of the Heart Association of Canada, and hundreds of private individuals who are now taking vitamin E for relief of their heart or circulatory symptoms. He begins his article with the story of a Huntsville, Ontario, wholesaler who had 33 friends all of whom had heart attacks. Twenty of them have been treated with vitamin E and are alive. Thirteen of them who were not treated with vitamin E are dead.

Hutton traces the story of the Shute Brothers' first interest in vitamin E when, in 1933, Evan Shute, M.D., an obstetrician, used it for the treatment of habitual abortion. He discovered that it appeared to delay the normal clotting of blood. He decided to use it on a patient suffering from purpura (bleeding) who could not be operated on because of a heart condition. Treatment with vitamin E helped the heart condition more than the purpura. Dr. Shute's brother, Wilfrid, who is also an M.D., soon joined forces with Dr. Evan in treating heart and circulatory patients with their own carefully-worked-out vitamin E therapy.

The mother of the two Shute Brothers was their next

[35]

heart patient. Mrs. Shute was so ill that she was unable to walk across the room. According to her own testimony she was gardening four weeks after she began to take vitamin E. Father C. A. MacKinnon testifies for vitamin E: "Phlebitis in my legs made me a bed case. The Shutes treated me with vitamin E and now I find that I can put in an average priest's day comfortably." Mary Salmond says, "Coronary thrombosis put me on my back for four months and I was told never to work again. After vitamin E treatment, I've been back at my job in a Toronto carpet plant for five years."

Shortly after the Shute Brothers began to use vitamin E in the treatment of heart disease, the governing body of all physicians and surgeons practicing in Ontario summoned them to give a report on their experience with vitamin E and heart disease. They presented the report. After spending two hours deliberating over the report, while they were at lunch, the Committee decided "on evidence submitted, the committee is convinced that vitamin E has no place in the treatment of cardiovascular (heart and blood vessel) disease." Apparently their decision was based on what they call faulty diagnosis. In other words, they imply that people cured by vitamin E did not really have serious heart trouble. The Shutes answer this with the statement that in 90 per cent of the cases that come to them they do not make the first diagnosis. Patients usually come to them after seeing one, two or three other doctors or specialists. In addition, the Shutes mention that two of the patients described in their report to the college of physicians and surgeons had been diagnosed as heart patients by physicians who were on the committee bringing in the report of incorrect diagnosis!

Medical Opposition to Vitamin E Therapy

Asked what is their own explanation for the medical opposition to the use of vitamin E, the Shutes admit that they do not know. "Some of our loudest critics are taking vitamin E themselves. Many dispense vitamin E but will not sign a prescription for it. Many doctors returned to practice on vitamin E, after coronaries disabled them, are ashamed to admit the source of their help, even to their closest friends."

Learning recently that enough vitamin E was being shipped to a certain hospital to supply dosage for about 16 people daily, they inquired whether some special tests were underway. They were told that no hospital patients were getting vitamin E. The full supply was for the personal use of staff physicians. The Shutes say that about 180 doctors and their families are among the 10,000 patients they have treated for heart and circulatory disease. The Shutes, who used to be meek and mild about criticism and neglect of their methods, have decided that it is necessary for them to fight for recognition of vitamin E, regardless of whose toes are trampled on or whose feelings are hurt in the process.

Vitamin E has been the subject of extensive debate in medical magazines in the United States and abroad. Yet in Montreal a businessman, put back on his feet

[37]

by the Shute treatment, decided to ask the Rotary Club to have Dr. Wilfrid Shute as a speaker. The chairman of the committee was a doctor who refused flatly to consider inviting Dr. Shute to speak. Later when a new committee was in charge, arrangements were made for Dr. Shute to speak before the Rotary and announcements were sent out. The reaction on the part of some medical members of the Rotary was instantaneous. They protested so strongly that the committee finally agreed not to cancel the speech, but to cancel the proposed broadcast of it. Later M.D. Rotarians tried to prevent the Montreal newspaper from publishing accounts of the speech. Mr. McConnell, the publisher of the *Star,* and members of his staff had benefited from being treated with vitamin E. So, in addition to defending freedom of the press, the *Star* editorial board was defending a friend whose integrity was unquestioned, when they published the following editorial:

"Montreal's reputation as a hospitable, courteous and open-minded city suffered, we fear, some damage as a result of the controversy inside the Rotary Club and now outside of it as well over the speech made this week by Dr. Wilfrid Shute. It is not a suitable thing—putting the case mildly—to invite a reputable man to Montreal to make a speech and then to take such steps as can be taken to restrict his audience and subject him to discourtesy. Far better to cancel the invitation altogether.

"Dr. Shute's address was the use of vitamin E in the treatment of heart disease. This is a topic of great

[38]

medical controversy, one upon which there are legitimate differences of opinion. But for some lamentable reason certain medical men feel so strongly that they are prepared to go to great lengths to prevent public discussion of it. This is not only unscientific, it also does no credit to a great and honorable profession which has done so much to push back the frontiers of medical knowledge. The advocates of the treatment in question are neither quacks nor charlatans, and in a free society, they are entitled to have their say.

"The Shute incident here is, unfortunately, not an isolated one in the record and history of medicine. Again and again the restless and enquiring mind has suffered slights and indignities at the hands of men who have refused to open new doors or even to walk through them when they have been opened by others."

In a survey done by Mr. Hutton among pharmaceutical houses who prepare vitamin E, he was told that in Toronto 28 per cent of the doctors use vitamin E and approve of its therapy, even though they will not indicate openly their approval. In a survey made by one company among 800 doctor customers, 228 made enthusiastic comments on the effectiveness of vitamin E in treating heart disease. Mr. Hutton goes on: "I spoke to an eminent physicist, a man largely responsible for a major Canadian contribution to the secret armament of World War II. He had personally found in vitamin E such a source of physical and mental endurance and efficiency that he had expressed the opinion that in a close war vitamin E supplied to key personnel might actually make the difference between

[39]

victory and defeat. I asked him if he would tell his story. He thought the matter over and then replied: 'No. I would like to, because it is truly remarkable. But somehow the medical profession has managed to give the idea that anyone who believes in vitamin E is— well, slightly in the screwball class. I just don't feel that I should expose myself to the inevitable comments if I speak openly'."

CHAPTER IV

Vitamin E Is a Powerful Preventive Agent

Dr. William Halden, University of Graz, Adviser on nutritional problems to the Austrian Government, Member of the Expert Panel on Nutrition of the World Health Organization. Member of the American Public Health Association.

The development of research work on vitamin E began with investigations by Dr. H. M. Evans and associates in California in 1922. A three-session symposium on vitamin E, organized by the late Sir Jack Drummond and Alfred Bacharach, took place in London, in April, 1939 when the course of further research on this remarkable vital element was outlined by distinguished scientists. After ten years, the second inter-

[41]

national congress on vitamin E was held in New York under the chairmanship of Dr. K. E. Mason of the Department of Anatomy, University of Rochester, New York. The long series of communications and discussions at that congress were published in the *Annals of the New York Academy of Medicine*. This volume contains a wealth of valuable information on vitamin E with many predictions on the future trend of research in this particular field.

The third international congress on vitamin E was held in Italy from September fifth to eighth in 1955 under very favorable auspices. More than 250 participants from all parts of the world attended the official inauguration and the subsequent sessions at the famous Ani Foundation on the beautiful island San Giorgio Maggiore, opposite the enchanting panorama of Venice.

The history of vitamin E has gone through various stages, the most interesting one, without a doubt, being the present one. It is characterized by the conviction that tocopherols (the name given the six different types of vitamin E, called by the Greek alphabet letters alpha, beta, gamma, delta, epsilon, zeta), are very helpful agents in preventive and curative medicine.

The first lectures on vitamin E and metabolic processes were given by Dr. P. L. Harris, Chief of Research Laboratories, D.P.I., Rochester, followed by a comprehensive report of Professor C. E. Mason of the University of Rochester. Dr. Harris outlined the situation in the field of present research, documenting his remarks with over one thousand references to medical

[42]

and scientific literature. One was astonished to learn from these and other American scientists about the wealth of biological and clinical information on this particular vitamin.

These findings would not have been possible without dependable analytical methods for determining the single tocopherols in natural sources of very intricate composition. It was chiefly the admirable work of Mary-Louise Quaife which decisively contributed to the knowledge of the occurrence of various types of tocopherols in natural foodstuffs. Some time ago Dr. Quaife married Dr. H. R. Bolliger of Basel, Switzerland. He gave a survey of the newest analytical methods and their use in the evaluation of tocopherols. Dr. Green from Vitamins, Ltd., Todworth, Surrey, England also made valuable contributions to this field. Then there were lectures by British, Danish, French, German, Italian, South American, Swiss and other researchers which were of special interest for the problems surrounding vitamin E and its relation to other vitamins, hormones and enzymes.

Most emphasis was given to the relation of vitamin E to the cardiovascular system (the heart and blood vessels) for of course there is great worldwide interest in this problem. There are very intimate connections between diet and circulation, especially from the standpoint of vitamin E administration, as was amply demonstrated in Venice.

Professor Henrik Dam of Copenhagen and his coworkers had found that the administration of large quantities of cod liver oil to experimental animals re-

[43]

sulted in severe disorders of the skin and other organs if the diet of these animals was devoid of vitamin E. All signs of illness disappeared in a rather short time after the supply of sufficient amounts of tocopherols or vitamin E.

The reason for this strange happening is the fact that cod liver oil contains highly-unsaturated fatty acids, like the group of acids that make up the so-called vitamin F. Such fatty acids make it easier for oxygen to go by way of the bloodstream to all cells, tissues and organs. You can easily understand, then, that these unsaturated fatty acids or vitamin F have great importance for the respiration or oxygenation of the most vital parts of our living.

The Danish investigators made another very important discovery in finding deposits of dark colored peroxides of fatty acids in the arteries at various parts of the animal body *if there was not sufficient vitamin E in the diet.* The occurrence of peroxides could be prevented by giving vitamin E or synthetic substances somewhat like vitamin E. One of these substances is methylene-blue which produces some effects similar to vitamin E, when it is given in appropriate, small quantities.

Here one can see the difference between a natural vital substance like vitamin E and a synthetic substance of the methylene-blue. When the supply of the methylene-blue was raised over a certain limit, very severe disorders occurred in the bodies of the laboratory animals, clearly showing the unbiological effect of such a substance. Vitamin E, however, can be supplied in

[44]

much higher doses than the usual ones without any undesirable reaction.

Take for instance some drug that may be given to you by a physician in a small dose, bringing you some comfort and help during a state of illness. If you should take the tenfold of such a poisonous agent it would badly harm you, and if you should take twenty times as much as the helpful dose it would probably kill you. In a similar way methylene-blue can be applied in small doses to experimental animals in order to prevent severe disturbances caused by an over-supply of highly unsaturated fatty acids. The ten- or twenty-fold doses would prove disastrous to the animals.

On the other hand, the natural tocopherols which are normal constituents of plants as well as animals and human beings may be applied in concentrations of many *milligrams* (as they are contained in every four ounces or so of many natural foodstuffs) daily for preventive purposes up to daily doses of *grams* (a thousand milligrams) without doing any harm. So, in other words, a thousand times as much vitamin E as you might get in food is not harmful, because it is a natural substance.

This fact has been emphasized by some researchers, especially Drs. Evan and Wilfrid Shute of the Shute Institute at London, Ontario, Canada. These scientists have already written in their papers on vitamin E in the treatment of hypertensive heart disease that the "dosage of alpha tocopherol varied with each type of heart disease and with each case within that type."

At the congress in Venice, Dr. Shute again described

[45]

a great many cases of successful treatment of cardio-vascular diseases with tocopherols, showing the results of this medication with dozens of marvelous colored pictures which made a deep impression on the audience.

The clinical results of the application of vitamin E on severe cases of cardiovascular and nervous diseases, degenerative muscular dystrophies and myopathies (muscle diseases) described by other scientists of international reputation clarified the importance of vitamin E as a valuable tool in practical medicine.

The history of vitamin E has gone through various stages, the most interesting one being without doubt the present one. It is characterized by the conviction that the tocopherols are very helpful as agents in preventive and curative medicine. The chief point of attack of tocopherols in the body seems to be intimately connected with the utilization of oxygen and therefore with cell respiration. As you know oxygen is absolutely essential for every process that goes on inside our bodies and it is believed that in many diseases one of the chief troubles is lack of enough oxygen in the cells.

The highly unsaturated fatty acids (such as vitamin F) act as biological "accelerators" of oxygen transport. In other words, they make it easier to move oxygen from place to place in the body. It is easy to understand that the process of oxygen-utilization can proceed too far and produce some unwelcome reactions. One of these might be the deposit of peroxides in the blood vessels and all of the disorders that might accompany such a state. In order to avoid this condition, nature provides "moderators" that prevent the overactivity of

[46]

all the various substances that promote the use of oxygen.

In the human body vitamin E plays this role of moderating, thus being able to counteract the too-rapid action of the other substances that are using up the oxygen. We might imagine it as a river in which the oxygen flows between two streams of those substances that accelerate and those that moderate like vitamin E. In this way the oxygen operates in the most effective manner, without going beyond the proper threshold, established by vitamin E. True respiration must be harmonized in order to make the best possible use of oxygen without forming any deposits in blood vessels. If vitamin E is continually supplied to the human body in appropriate quantities as they occur in natural food-stuffs like wheat germ and whole grains, almonds, nuts, oilseeds and oils pressed therefrom, then the most economical conditions for a normal circulation prevail.

Vitamin E and its natural sources are of course not the only requisites for a normal circulation and condition of blood vessels. Some authors are of the opinion, expressed also at the International Congress in Venice, that some vitamins of the B group as well as vitamins A and C form an auxiliary team of vital substances that help to accomplish the manifold roles the toco-pherols have got to play in the concert of vitamins, that accompanies the biological harmony of a well-balanced respiration, heart action and easy-going circulation.

CHAPTER V

When Doctors Prescribe Vitamin E

Vitamin E used by normally healthy people as a preventive of heart disease and in the maintenance of general good health is safe in almost any amount, particularly the ordinary 100 or 200 mg. dosage most people use. In cases of serious heart disease its effective use is trickier. Still, in the hands of a competent physician, vitamin E often achieves success where orthodox medications may have failed miserably. Its proper use is a technique no intelligent, conscientious physician can afford to ignore.

When a doctor first decides to use vitamin E in treating heart ailments he runs smack into the problem of dosage. Too little and he becomes disillusioned about vitamin E's powers. If enormous amounts are prescribed in certain cases, the results may be equally unsatisfactory.

Drs. Wilbur and Evan Shute have been treating cardiac patients with vitamin E for nearly 22 years. They have personally cared for or supervised the treatment of more than 29,000 cardiovascular patients. The fruits of their experience, as presented in *The Summary* (December, 1967), offer welcome guidelines for physicians new to vitamin E therapy. The Shutes believe, "The key to success depends upon fitting the dosage to the individual patient's peculiar requirements. Different forms of cardiovascular disease require different ranges of effective dosage. For example, coronary artery insufficiency, whatever the underlying pathology, usually responds to between 800 and 1200 mg. of alpha tocopherol (vitamin E) daily. However, an occasional patient may need much more."

Six Weeks for Results

To get specific, the doctors discuss the use of vitamin E in treating the painful angina pectoris that often follows effort or excitement. These patients are checked for any other cardiac complications; if none shows up they are put on 800 mg. alpha tocopherol daily for six weeks. It takes five to ten days before symptoms are relieved or diminished to the point the patient and the physician can tell it. But after six weeks, the Shutes expect definite response. Then no matter how good the results, the patient stays on the 800 mg. daily indefinitely. If he stops, he can lose all he gained within three to seven days. Lessening the dosage will lead to a slower but still certain return of the symptoms.

If the angina patient has an elevated blood pressure, the Shutes combine the 800 mg. dosage with a tranquilizer for about six weeks. By then the blood pressure is usually lowered and can be satisfactorily controlled by the vitamin E, without drugs.

In cases of acute coronary occlusion (heart attack) the Shutes say 1600 mg. of alpha tocopherol a day should be started immediately by the attending physician. Although a smaller dose might be adequate in most cases, they believe it is best to make sure the maximum help is being given. In these cases the oxygen-conserving power of alpha tocopherol, along with its ability to dilate the capillaries, can be a major factor in saving the heart. The infarct itself can be greatly reduced in size, and damage to adjacent tissues may also be prevented. But if strong vitamin E therapy is postponed, it may soon be too late to prevent serious tissue damage. Lowering the oxygen need of the laboring heart, as vitamin E does, adds to the chances of survival.

Ideal Test

The Shutes call these acute coronary occlusions "ideal test problems" because they give alpha tocopherol a chance to show what it really can do. The electrocardiogram markings made by acute coronary occlusion are always typical, but when the patient begins using vitamin E, the changes are diminished, and, "the recovery of the electrocardiogram is more rapid and complete than it is without alpha tocopherol . . ."

It is expected that most of the heart attack victims seen by the Shutes come weeks, months, or even years after the attack. "If cardiologists really believe that a

[50]

majority of patients regain good or near normal health following an occlusion they are mistaken . . . ," say the Shutes. "The majority of those we have seen have had a definite and usually marked abnormality of the electrocardiogram. . ." The Shutes look to the pulse rate and cardiogram changes for guidance in determining adequate dosage and adequate protection. These patients suffer areas of decreasing injury that fan out from the basic hurt itself. When such a patient is treated with vitamin E the zone of injury may lessen and so may the radiating areas of damage, as reflected by changes in the electrocardiogram. This hopeful sequence is news to old-time cardiologists, "because it so rarely occurred in their experience before the days of alpha tocopherol."

Heart attack patients appear to respond more rapidly and completely to vitamin E therapy than patients with other types of heart disease. Ordinarily, they are started on 800 mg. a day with increases of 200 to 400 mg. a day at six week intervals until some improvement is seen.

Signs of acute rheumatic fever may last for only as little as 3 to 7 days and rarely longer than 3 or 4 weeks. But as soon as they appear, the Shutes urge immediate use of the full dosage; 600 mg. of vitamin E daily by mouth, regardless of age. In cases of continuing rheumatic fever, ". . . If we can send the patient to the hospital and have full laboratory and other facilities for treatment we give a trial of full dosage since here we are able to detect adverse responses as soon as they occur. . . ." But most chronic rheumatic fever patients are treated cautiously; 90 mg. a day for the first four

[51]

weeks, 120 mg. for the second four weeks; and 150 mg. for the third four weeks. Usually 150 mg. turns out to be the maximum safe level.

The "Despair" Cases

Chronic rheumatic heart disease is the despair of most cardiac specialists. These patients have congestive failure, auricular fibrillation and can take almost no exercise whatsoever. "Yet we have had patients in this category who had spent 6 to 19 months in bed under classical therapy, who were able to resume full activity and maintain normal living with increasing strength. This has occurred in as little as a month on alpha tocopherol treatment. . . ."

One patient the Shutes tell about has done her housework for the last four years on 150 mg. of vitamin E a day, even though she was told by a very competent heart specialist that she would never be able to do another bit of work of any kind. When this patient tried to increase her dosage to 180 mg. a day she got dizzy. When she reduced it to 120, the symptoms of her heart trouble returned.

All of these warnings and precautionary measures pertain to unusual heart conditions: "A patient with a normal or low blood pressure and with no evidence of congestive failure can usually, but not quite always, tolerate any quantity of alpha tocopherol. . . . Like digitalis and insulin and thyroid extract, the right dose is the dose that begins to show definite improvement, in four to six weeks in this case. The maintenance dose is the same. . . ."

[52]

Part Two:

THE CHOLESTEROL-
HEART DISEASE
RELATIONSHIP

CHAPTER VI

How Heart Attacks Were Prevented by the "Prudent Diet"

You, like 1,000 volunteers in a recently concluded experiment, can prove to yourself that a good, reasonable diet is an excellent way to avoid heart disease. The test was designed and directed by Norman Jolliffe, M.D., head of New York City's Bureau of Nutrition. His now-famous *Prudent Diet* is given credit for reducing the number of heart attacks in healthy middle-aged men to 60 to 80 per cent below that which is ordinarily to be expected.

The volunteers led normal lives, except that they agreed to purchase only certain foods and to prepare them in certain ways. There were no drugs whatsoever

[55]

involved in the experiment. The men were free to continue their lives with no other changes. They even continued to smoke with no objection. Every 10 weeks they met for a panel discussion with doctors, both as a means of maintaining the interest of the subjects in the experiment, and also to allow the doctors to keep track of the progress of the experiment.

The heart-health of a similar group of men living in Framingham, Massachusetts, served as a comparison for the results of the Prudent Diet. The men were tested by U.S. Public Health Service doctors for cholesterol accumulations in the blood, just as the New Yorkers who figured in the experiment were tested by Dr. Jolliffe's assistants. Various circumstances of health (overweight, high cholesterol levels, physical heart and circulatory imperfections, etc.) were also considered, as an additional risk likely to lead to heart attack.

Among those with one of the risk factors in their background, Framingham men had nearly 20 heart attacks per 1,000 men, while the Prudent Diet group had a rate of about 5 per 1,000 men. However, the true value of the diet was dramatized by those having more than one risk factor. The Framingham men showed the expected increase in the number of heart attacks—their score: 36 per 1,000 men. The men on the diet not only avoided an increase, but actually decreased their likelihood of suffering a heart attack—their score: less than 2 per 1,000 men. The *Prudent Diet* was the only controlled element of difference between the 2 groups of men.

Essentially the diet reduced the consumption of satu-

[56]

rated fats, which are contained in such things as butter, whole milk cheeses, margarines, eggs and meats such as beef, pork and lamb. Instead the men ate foods relatively high in unsaturated fatty acids, such as corn oil, fish, nuts, and grains, plus lean meats such as poultry and veal. The result was a remarkable and consistent lowering of cholesterol levels in every grouping of the cases.

Three groups were made of the subjects according to their original cholesterol-level readings. In one group, which averaged 307 milligrams per milliliter, 10 weeks on the Prudent Diet brought the reading down to 260. The second group dropped from 257 to 219, and the third group went from 207 to 189—all as the result of nothing other than 10 weeks on the *Prudent Diet.*

People are moved to wonder how painful it must be to stay on a diet as effective as all that. Actually, most people would find such a diet quite satisfying and quite appetizing. Equally important, it is possible to maintain such a diet indefinitely. Here, for example, is a sample day's menu:

Breakfast:
>4 ounces fruit juice or tomato juice, strawberries or melon in season.
>1 egg or 2 ounces of cottage cheese
>1 slice of bread

Lunch or Supper:
>4 ounces of fish or seafood, or poultry or lean meat

[57]

12½ calorie value vegetable (all you want)
2 slices bread
1 serving fruit

Dinner:

8 ounces fish or poultry or meat
1 portion 25 calorie vegetable
12½ calorie vegetable (all you want)
1 slice bread
1 serving fruit, 75 calories

Between Meals:

2 glasses skim milk
3 servings of fruit or fruit juice—75 calories each

The diet's footnotes specify that no more than 4 eggs per week should be eaten, that fish should be part of at least 3 lunches and 2 dinners per week, and only one lunch a week should comprise the leaner cuts of beef, lamb, pork or veal. We presume that the item designated as 12½ calorie value vegetable is a salad of green, and the recommended dressing is simply vinegar or lemon juice.

The reason for the name, *The Prudent Diet,* is obvious. There is nothing faddish about this selection, no problem of near-starvation. It is a sensible diet and one that can be maintained as long as one is interested in eating properly.

There are several items suggested by Dr. Jolliffe to which we take exception, but the diet is so far superior to most diets one sees that we hesitate to discourage its use. We would, however, substitute some other beverage for milk, of course. Bread would be eliminated too,

[58]

and perhaps baked potato substituted at lunch or dinner. We would say 2 eggs at breakfast, and no cottage cheese. Calorie counting, we believe, is unnecessary when the foods that are eaten are fresh, unadulterated and sensibly prepared.

Eggs are limited in the *Prudent Diet* because of their cholesterol content. We believe that such limitation is unnecessary because eggs also contain lecithin in relatively large amounts, and lecithin is an excellent aid to the body in making proper use of cholesterol. A test at Alameda County Hospital showed eggs to be less of a villain than their bad publicity indicates. Adelle Davis (*Let's Eat Right to Keep Fit,* Harcourt, Brace & World, Inc., N.Y.C.) tells of patients at that hospital who were given fat from egg yolks equivalent to 36 eggs. In no case did the cholesterol level of the blood rise above its original reading. Aside from the lecithin value in eggs, one should bear in mind the heavy concentration of B vitamins they hold, and these have also demonstrated their value in controlling cholesterol levels.

The ability of lecithin to help in the proper metabolism of cholesterol is too often neglected by those who write about the cholesterol problem. Lecithin occurs in fat-rich natural foods. One of its main effects is the breaking of cholesterol into much smaller particles. These are easily transported in the blood stream with no tendency to pile up or stick to the walls of the arteries. They can be absorbed easily by the tissues and the cholesterol "problem" is eliminated.

(Many fats taken into the system do not come

[59]

equipped with lecithin. Hydrogenated fat-containing foods are particularly cited, and these are the very ones which are highest in cholesterol. These are also the ones, logically enough, which make up a large part of the diet of many Americans, Americans who have been shown to have one of the world's highest scores for coronary death rate.)

We believe that one should make a special effort to take advantage of lecithin's properties to maintain a healthy cholesterol level. By this we mean that lecithin-rich foods should be eaten frequently to compensate for ordinary fat intake of all kinds. Lecithin is generously contained in the natural vegetable oils. These are also rich in unsaturated fats, the fats rated so important in anti-cholesterol eating.

Why Unsaturated Fats?

The term "unsaturated fats" sounds familiar because we hear it so frequently, but there is no doubt that people are frightened by the technical sound of it. Just what does it mean? Fatty acids occur in all sorts of series. They are shaped like a chain, to the eye of a biochemist. Some of the links are open on these chains, allowing for the entrance of a new substance. Others are solidly closed.

The open chains are the unsaturated (unfilled) fats. When they enter the body, the opening they have allows for the entrance of, and combining with, some body substance or other, and this combination allows for a new use of the fat in the body, an easy absorption. A saturated fat can combine with nothing in the body

[60]

and must be absorbed or eliminated as is. This is where the problem occurs. When the body is not ready or able to absorb a saturated fat, the fat wanders aimlessly in the blood stream and can pile up and clog the passages.

In some cases processing makes saturated fats out of unsaturated fats. This is called hydrogenation. Hydrogenated fats are those in which hydrogen is forced to take up the opening in the link of the unsaturated fat series. Oftentimes oxygen would normally take it up, and oxygen can cause a rancidity in the fat. Hydrogenated fats don't get rancid, but hydrogenated fats are a real problem for the body to cope with. Liquid fats are more healthful and just as useful and tasty.

We are pleased to have Dr. Jolliffe's evidence which demonstrates the value of a sensible selection of foods in preventing heart trouble. It reinforces arguments that we have been presenting for more than ten years. We believe that most chronic diseases result directly from poor food selection which, in turn, encourages poor metabolism of essential nutrients. Eat fresh, simple foods, and your body will make good use of them. More processing means more problems. Don't try to avoid cholesterol-containing foods—you can't, if you hope to maintain good nutritional balance. Cholesterol is in all animal-originated foods. Instead eat foods that will provide the ammunition for a good defense against any dangerous cholesterol accumulation. These are foods high in lecithin and unsaturated fats.

[61]

CHAPTER VII

Vitamin C Battles Excess Cholesterol

Heart disease is most commonly caused by atherosclerosis, or hardening of the arteries. Actually, the "hardening" is caused by fatty cholesterol deposits which build up on the artery walls and narrow the passageways the blood must pass through. When this happens to the major arteries that lead to the heart, slowing down the flow during an emergency or some strenuous activity when the blood need increases, it causes heart symptoms, including angina pectoris— severe chest pains. It can lead to heart attack and death.

The Fifth International Convention on Dietary Lipids meeting in October, 1966, heard encouraging testimony by Dr. Emil Ginter, chief of the biochemistry department, Institute of Nutritional Research, Bratislava, Czechoslovakia, that vitamin C can combat the development of atherosclerosis. In his experiments he fed a cholesterol-rich diet to laboratory pigs, but added a daily supplement of 50 milligrams of vitamin C. Then he sacrificed the animals and measured the cholesterol accumulation in the brain, liver, stomach and the main artery of the heart. He found that the cholesterol deposits were 30 to 40 per cent lower than in control guinea pigs fed the same cholesterol-rich diet, with only 5 milligrams of supplementary vitamin C.

To check the vitamin C-cholesterol relationship further, a new group of guinea pigs were fed a diet completely free of ascorbic acid for two weeks. Then a normal diet was introduced, with .5 milligrams of supplementary vitamin C administered orally every day. The 30 control animals were fed the same normal diet, but received ten times as much vitamin C. After a year, cholesterol accumulation in the liver, adrenals, brain and other tissues, including the wall of the main heart artery, were 30 per cent greater in the animals on .5 milligrams of vitamin C than in the better-nourished controls.

The *American Journal of Physiology* (December, 1950) described work done at Harvard University, Washington, D.C., with high cholesterol dogs.

These researchers found that, in dogs, excess cholesterol reduces the amount of vitamin C in the blood. The more cholesterol the dogs received the greater the vitamin C they lost in their urine. In other words,

[63]

high cholesterol levels create a vitamin C deficiency. We know now that the converse is also true, namely, increasing vitamin C reduces excess cholesterol.

In 1961 an article by W. J. McCormick, M.D., stated, "Regarding the nutritional habits of the coronary thrombosis group, it was found that as a whole there was a marked tendency to deficient intake of the B and C vitamins, in that nearly all were predominantly white bread users and low in their use of fresh fruits and salads." Dr. McCormick went on to say that a deficiency of the B and C vitamins may result in liver damage so that normal amounts of cholesterol cannot be assimilated by the body. Patients afflicted with abnormally high cholesterol count are sometimes advised by their physicians not to eat liver, eggs and other cholesterol-rich foods. On the other hand, in patients given a diet that contains ample B vitamins and C, and then given desiccated or cooked whole liver, there is usually a dramatic decrease in the blood cholesterol, in spite of a larger intake.

To get back to the work of Dr. Ginter, he told his convention audience about a survey conducted by the Czechs, involving 1,000 school children. It revealed that 97 per cent suffered from vitamin C lack during the winter and spring, when C-rich fruits and vegetables are less abundant. Notably, there was corresponding rise in cholesterol levels in the winter.

As Dr. Ginter stated in his report, the main trouble we have with cholesterol is in the difficulty certain bodies have in using it up. Responsible scientists have aimed their efforts at finding a way of helping the body

[64]

process its cholesterol supply, so that troublesome residues will not collect in the bloodstream. One way to accomplish this is by eating foods rich in nutrients known to help the body handle cholesterol; another is by activating the natural equipment the body has for using cholesterol properly.

Perhaps you eat candy which depletes cholesterol-reducing vitamin B in the body. Do you smoke? It costs you vitamin C. If only for its effect on cholesterol metabolism, this vitamin is too precious to be dissipated unnecessarily.

Part Three:

CARBOHYDRATES AND THE HEART

CHAPTER VIII

Sugar Taxes Your Heart

Some two million people will die in the United States this year, according to estimates based on figures from the National Office of Vital Statistics. More than half of those, a full million, will die as a result of arteriosclerosis (hardening of the arteries) and hypertension (high blood pressure). Of this unfortunate million, there is reason to believe, at least half will have developed atherosclerosis, the condition leading to their deaths, because of too much sugar in their diets.

That is the inevitable conclusion that must be drawn from two studies published in *The Lancet* by Professor John Yudkin of the University of London, one of the world's leading nutritionists and a man whose profound knowledge leaves him appalled at what modern civilization is doing to its citizens.

It was a highly appropriate coincidence that Profes-

[69]

sor Yudkin, an independent scientist who refuses to be hidebound by the consensus of medical opinion, exploded his bombshell in *The Lancet* on Independence Day, July 4, 1964. In it he pointed out the very strong reasons that exist for believing that the medical profession has been on the wrong track in trying to connect heart disease with the amount of fat consumed in the diet. Even though the American Heart Association has now gone on record as advocating reduction in dietary fats for the prevention of heart disease, the fact remains that in ten years of intensive work by thousands of qualified investigators, nobody has ever succeeded in proving that there is any cause-and-effect relationship between dietary fat and atherosclerosis, the leading cause of heart disease. It is true that atherosclerosis (the most prevalent form of arteriosclerosis) is characterized by deposits of cholesterol in the arteries. This has been demonstrated beyond any reasonable doubt. But is it these cholesterol deposits that cause the eventual failure of the heart from ischemic heart disease (failure of the blood supply to the heart) and are the cholesterol deposits caused by consumption of cholesterol in the diet? Neither of these two questions has ever been satisfactorily answered.

As an example of the type of contradiction into which investigators have run, a recent study of A. S. Loginov published in the Russian heart journal *Kardiologiya* (2, 1, 1962) was a compilation of statistics concerned with the North African country, Ethiopia. It was shown that diet in Ethiopia does affect the blood serum level of cholesterol, but that whether the serum

[70]

level is high or low, there is practically no heart disease in that country. A. M. Cohen reported in the *American Heart Journal* (65, 291, 1963) that Jews living in Yemen eat very high fat diets yet have little heart disease, whereas those of the same national strain who have migrated to Israel where they eat a more "civilized" and less primitive diet, show the same tendency to contract atherosclerosis as is noticeable in Western Europe and the United States.

Other studies have shown that while many victims of atherosclerosis and ischemic heart disease have high levels of serum cholesterol, there are others who do not. And equally puzzling has been the fact that very large portions of our population show high serum cholesterol on testing, yet never develop heart or circulatory diseases. For these reasons, the American Medical Association and the FDA have never been willing to give unqualified endorsement to the idea that you can prevent a heart attack by reducing the amount of cholesterol in your diet.

Since 1957, Professor Yudkin has been not only pointing out these discrepancies that cast doubt on the cholesterol theory, but he has also offered an alternative theory that the medical profession has been doing its best to ignore. It is true, said Dr. Yudkin, that we can show statistically that a large proportion of people who get heart attacks eat a diet high in fats. But all that this proves is that there is an association between the two elements, whereas a cause-and-effect relationship has proven impossible to demonstrate. What is more, a high fat diet is nothing new in human history. As far

[71]

back as our knowledge of mankind goes, people who could afford to do so have always eaten large quantities of meat with the fat that goes along with it. Why, then, should the incidence of heart disease increase so sharply in modern times, and keep growing from one year to the next? Why didn't our ancestors a thousand years ago drop on all sides of heart disease, since there was just as much fat in their diets as in ours?

Dr. Yudkin's answer is that the cause is not fat but sugar.

Quoting studies made by the Food and Agriculture Organization of the United Nations, he points out that while it is true that fat consumption increases as countries and their populations grow wealthier, sugar consumption increases with it and at an even faster rate. "Intakes of fat and sugar . . . not only rise by the same high factor of about four-fold from the poorest group of countries to the wealthiest group but are almost exactly the same in absolute quantities. (However) the relative constancy of carbohydrate intake with increase in income hides an increase in sugar intake, which almost exactly matches the fall in other carbohydrate, mostly starch."

In other words, the consumption of fat and of carbohydrate increase at just about the same rate with an increase in the means to buy them. However, with the carbohydrate group the consumption of sugars increased. This indicates, as shown by Dr. Yudkin in a chart derived from statistics from 41 countries, that of all foods, it is sugar that has the fastest increasing rate of consumption in the wealthier countries where the

[72]

rate of deaths by heart disease keeps increasing at an equally fast rate. And it is just as reasonable to suppose that the increase in heart disease is due to the increased intake of sugar as it is to suppose it is because of more fat in the diet.

The reason why most investigators have concentrated on the fat is primarily because the sugar intake is more masked. Sugar is added to most processed foods today, from a can of tomatoes to a package of frozen chicken a la king, because it adds palatability to the sterilized and flavorless messes today's food manufacturers sell for popular consumption. Thus it is very hard to make an estimate of how much sugar we are actually consuming, whereas the intake of fat is far more obvious.

Your doctor might be very surprised to learn that the average per capita consumption of sugar in this country is more than half a pound a day. He knows that even a quarter pound a day is far, far too much, and given any idea of how high a given patient's sugar consumption may be, he would probably try to reduce it. But even with sincere and strenuous efforts, it would be virtually impossible for the average person eating an average diet of processed foods to reduce his sugar consumption to a proper level. Even if he eliminates all sweet drinks and desserts, there remain fantastic quantities of the sweet poison in practically every food that has had anything to do with the factory before reaching the consumer. Dr. Yudkin estimates that a full 50 per cent of the sugar consumption of the average individual, which is to say roughly a quarter pound a

[73]

day, is derived from sugar added in food processing that you may not even know you are eating.

Nevertheless, that leaves the other 50 per cent which you yourself add to your diet if you are so ill-advised as to be a user of refined sugar. And the fact that some people use sugar without any heed of consequences while others attempt to eliminate sugar as much as they possibly can, leaves scope for tremendous variation in the individual consumption of sugar. If the per capita figure is half a pound a day, we can say with confidence that there are many people who eat a quarter pound or less of sugar daily, and many others who may consume a pound or more every day of their lives. It is precisely on this question of individual variation that the cholesterol theory of the causation of heart disease is at its weakest. Statistically, analyzing a large group of people or an entire population, you can show that as cholesterol in the diet increases, so does heart disease. But when it comes to examining the individuals who actually suffer from heart disease, it has proven impossible to pin down a definite relationship.

Startling Statistics

Dr. Yudkin has subjected his theory to the very same test, but with vastly different results. He studied two groups of London Hospital patients. The first group consisted of those who had been admitted to the hospital for either a recent heart attack or an atherosclerotic condition. The second group consisted of those admitted for accidental injuries who, except for the

[74]

accidents they had suffered, could be said to be in good health and were not known to have any kind of difficulties concerning the heart or circulatory system. The second group was to be studied as a control, to be contrasted with group one.

What Dr. Yudkin found was that *without exception* the hospital patients with arterial disease were consuming substantially more sugar than those in the control group. On the average they were consuming twice as much. Even more remarkable as a confirmation, it was found that "in patients with peripheral arterial disease, more detailed analysis suggests that the degree of atherosclerosis was proportional to the amount of dietary sugar." In other words, it was possible to do in this single study what could not be done in 10 years of studying the possible relationship between fat consumption and atherosclerosis. It was possible to show statistically that not only is the atherosclerotic a heavy user of sugar, but the more sugar he uses the worse is his atherosclerotic condition.

Most remarkable of all, it was found so uniformly and without exception that the sufferer from atherosclerosis is a user of unusually large amounts of sugar, that even a small number of samples produced a statistically significant correlation.

Here's how that works. Suppose you want to find out whether there is a relationship between two elements —let's say, wearing brown shoes and being a good walker. You take a hundred good walkers and see how many of them wear brown shoes. If you find that 60 wear brown shoes and 40 wear black, this may or

[75]

may not be of some significance. You then have to examine a thousand good walkers or ten thousand or a hundred thousand until you reach a point where it becomes mathematically inescapable that the two factors either are or are not related. But if among your randomly selected 100 good walkers, you find that every single one of them wears brown shoes, then you know immediately that there is a significant relationship. It can no longer be the result of sheer coincidence or accident.

And it is for precisely this same reason that Professor Yudkin's study, even though a small one, is a highly significant one. The chance that the relationship he has shown between high sugar consumption and atherosclerosis could occur accidentally is computed to be less than one in two thousand. This brings it very close to certainty that eating large amounts of sugar is a prime cause, if not the only cause, of the disease that kills more of us than any other and is far and away responsible for more deaths in middle age than is any other.

Our ancestors a hundred years ago ate perhaps two pounds of sugar a year. This is practically no sugar at all, yet they could work harder for longer hours, think loftier and clearer thoughts, raise larger families and in every way demonstrate very high energy levels. You don't need sugar for energy. It is nothing but sweet poison that begins attacking a person's teeth the moment it enters the mouth and never stops attacking somewhere as long as it remains in the system.

[76]

They say the price of sugar is rising. If we could get it free, the price would still be too high.

Experimental Evidence

Further corroboration that sugar is a major cause of heart disease has been appearing fast in England, recently in an article in *The Lancet,* December 24, 1966.

Dr. K. J. Kingsbury of St. Mary's Hospital conducted an extensive study in which 338 male, atherosclerotic patients were chosen, at random from a group of mixed social, economic, and occupational classes. These patients were from various parts of the country, but the majority of them hailed from the Greater London area. They were investigated clinically, arteriographically, and with a standard series of biochemical tests, whereupon they were then admitted to a follow-up system.

These non-diabetic, atherosclerotic men with claudication (arterial obstruction) were classified into three groups of arterial disease — slight, moderate, and extensive.

Making an analysis of all three groups of patients and subjects, the doctors found that the greater the degree of atherosclerosis present, the less is the ability of the patient to metabolize glucose.

Dr. Kingsbury attempted to determine whether either the age or the degree of sickness of the patient could cause the lowered tolerance to sugar, but got only negative results. He concluded that the reverse is true

[77]

—it is the intolerance to glucose that causes the athero-sclerosis.

Seventy men were chosen for this study and were then divided into three groups. The first group con-sisted of 20 men who had suffered a coronary attack during the previous three weeks; the second group con-sisted of 25 men with arterial disease of the legs; and the third group consisted of 25 healthy men whose ages ranged from 45 to 66 years of age.

The results of this study are astounding! The coro-nary patients daily consumed an average of 132 grams of sugar, the arterial disease group consumed 141 grams —the healthy group 77 grams. The difference in results between the first two groups and the third group is so great that it is almost impossible for it to have occurred by chance.

Dr. Yudkin also pointed out that "There is un-doubtedly a genetic factor as well as an environmental factor involved in this heart disease." He stated that there were certain families who suffered an unusually high incidence of coronary heart disease—possibly because their members shared similar factors such as an excess of cholesterol in the blood, a heavy cigarette smoking experience, diabetes mellitus, or perhaps even hypertension. He stated that he was quite uncertain as to whether there was a basic genetic predisposition to coronary heart disease.

A most interesting study appeared in the *American Heart Journal,* (vol. 45, 1953), concerning two Israeli tribes, the Yemenites and the Bedouin. Dr. Fritz Drey-fuss conducted this study and pointed out that the

[78]

Yemenites, in particular, seemed to be immune to coronary arteriosclerosis! He had first observed this phenomenon in the medical wards of Hadassah-Hebrew University and later gathered statistics from all over Israel. He then studied with Dr. Joannes Groen, head of the Medical Center's Department of Internal Medicine, and found that the Bedouin, a roving desert tribe, were also almost completely free of this common type of heart disease. After intensive research, the doctors felt sure that the answer to the tribe's immunity must lie in some dietary factor.

Sugar Undermined Health

It was observed that the Yemenites who had recently arrived in Israel were almost entirely free of diabetes, whereas the Yemenites of the same age who had lived in Israel for more than 25 years suffered from diabetes just as frequently as the other peoples from the Western countries.

The Yemenites who suffered from diabetes were also the victims of arteriosclerotic complications such as heart disease. It seemed quite probable that a change in some environmental factor, operating over the course of many years, was responsible for this diabetes accompanied by cardiac complications.

The results of the dietary investigations were unbelievable! The most significant change in the diet of the Yemenites upon their arrival in Israel was the fact that while living in Yemen, they consumed their carbohydrates in the form of starch—such as potatoes and bread. Upon their arrival in Israel, about one-third of their starch was replaced with sugar, which had been an almost non-existent part of their diet in Yemen.

The same held true for the Bedouin, whose diet was almost identical to that of the Yemenites. Dr. Dreyfuss and his associates then concluded that *"sugar* seemed to be the dietary villain leading to the development of diabetes, arteriosclerosis and heart disease."

Another study was conducted over a six-year period by Dr. Thomas Francis, Jr. and his associates at the University of Michigan Medical School. The study was carried out in Tecumseh, Michigan, a small city with a population of approximately 9,500 people. Dr. Francis found that an elevated blood sugar level was indeed a strong indicator of a future heart attack—much stronger, in fact, than blood fats and high blood pressure, two factors which now are most commonly linked with heart disease.

Consumption Keeps Growing

In the world as a whole, the consumption of sugar in the past 25 years has more than doubled. It has been recently shown that in the United States during the last 70 years, the consumption of fats has only increased by 12 per cent. There has also been a significant increase in the ratio of the polyunsaturated fats to the more dangerous saturated fats. With such a low percentage relating to the consumption of fats, coronary heart disease should show a marked decline, instead of the very considerable rise that has in fact occurred if fat were the chief cause. However, during the same

[80]

period, sugar consumption has increased by 120 per cent! Heart disease has increased proportionately.

It has been observed that men who have developed coronary heart disease have been eating diets not differing quantitatively or qualitatively in the fat content as compared to men who did not develop the disease. On the other hand, there is evidence now relating the fact that men who have recently experienced a myocardial infarction have been eating twice as much sugar as those men who manifested no evidence of coronary heart disease. This difference is highly significant and of the utmost importance.

So, whether it's a piece of cake, a candy bar, or the sweetening used on cereals, sugars play a more important role in the ill health of a typical American diet —more important, in fact, than the fats he eats. With such an abundance of evidence linking sugar and coronary heart disease, one should be fully aware of its consequences and try to eliminate sugar from the diet entirely.

CHAPTER IX

Carbohydrate Controls Cholesterol

One of the most important of recent studies was published in the November, 1967 *American Journal of Clinical Nutrition* by the very well known nutritionists of the University of Iowa, Willard A. Krehl, M.D., Robert E. Hodges, M.D., and two associates, Alfredo Lopez-S, and Eleanor I. Good. After reviewing the dietary habits and heart disease death rates of people living in western countries, this group of expert nutritionists has confirmed that the type of carbohydrate eaten is basic in the development of atherosclerotic heart disease. The overall amount has changed little in recent years, they point out, but there has been a significant switch away from consumption of complex carbohydrates—the starches of such foods as cereals, potatoes and vegetables—and an increase in the intake of simple carbohydrates such as refined sugar and the foods that contain it like syrups and sweets.

In the recent book *Diet and Disease* by Drs. Cheraskin, Ringsdorf and Clark of the University of Alabama, the even more positive conclusion is drawn that the eating in any quantity of simple carbohydrates such as refined sugar increases the blood cholesterol level significantly, while the eating of complex carbohydrates such as potatoes actually *reduces* the amount of cholesterol in the blood.

All would seem to lead to the conclusion that anyone troubled with a high level of blood cholesterol could not do better for himself than immediately to eliminate all sugar from his diet.

The Iowa nutritionists cite their study of the relationship between the heart disease death rate and food intake trend in 15 European countries. During the period 1948-1959, there was an increase in the consumption of simple carbohydrates and fat in those countries, while the amount of complex carbohydrates consumed decreased. Although the researchers found no appreciable change in the consumption of protein, the amount of complex carbohydrate decreased from 306 to 268 grams, and the consumption of simple carbohydrate increased from 113 to 135 grams. "Evidently, affluent societies relish diets containing substantial amounts of fats and are also partial to sweets and to free sugar. This hypothesis was confirmed by the present study in which close relationships between

[83]

simple carbohydrate consumption and fat consumption were established . . . ," the Iowa researchers reported.

The survey of Austria, Belgium, Denmark, Finland, France, Germany, Greece, Ireland, Italy, Netherlands, Norway, Portugal, Switzerland, Sweden and the United Kingdom also showed that the mortality rate from atherosclerotic heart disease increased in the 1948 to 1959 decade. The researchers indicated that the death rate increased as the per cent of calories derived from simple sugars increased. For example, in France the annual consumption of sugar in 1950 was 22.8 kilograms per capita and in 1962, 29.6 kilograms. At the same time, the death rate (per 100,000) increased from 219 to 222, the Iowa researchers reported. A similar pattern was noted in the other countries studied.

In February, 1967 the Iowa scientists wrote in the *American Journal of Clinical Nutrition* that the carbohydrates in the diet may be just as capable as saturated fats of pushing up the cholesterol level of the blood. "As the amount of sucrose (refined sugar, jams, jellies, syrup, milk and fruits) is increased and the quantity of complex carbohydrates (cereals, potatoes and flour) decreased the concentration of cholesterol and more particularly triglycerides rises." A survey of 16 countries conducted by the Interdepartmental Committee on Nutrition For National Development showed that countries having the highest cholesterol values also ranked first in the consumption of simple sugar, they reported.

Related to the Iowa findings is Dr. Henry A. Schroeder's research indicating that variations in the amounts

[84]

of the trace elements cadmium and chromium in the body may provide a clue to the cause of cardiovascular diseases. Too much cadmium may trigger high blood pressure, while high levels of chromium may act as a protective agent. According to Dr. Schroeder, eating large amounts of sugar upsets that balance. The more sugar a person consumes, the greater is the body's metabolic demand for chromium. Adding to the problem is the fact that the refining of sugar removes chromium, Dr. Schroeder explained.

The Iowa nutritionists studied the relationship between the heart disease death rate and food intake in 15 European countries, and found that the mortality rate from atherosclerotic heart disease increased as the per cent of calories derived from simple sugars increased. In France the annual consumption of sugar in 1950 was 22.8 kilograms per capita, and in 1962, 29.6 kilograms. At the same time the death rate increased from 219 to 222 per 100,000. The pattern was repeated in the other countries studied.

It was ten years ago that *Prevention* discovered and described a rather obscure book, *How to Prevent Heart Attacks* by Benjamin P. Sandler, M.D. We then characterized the book as "so revolutionary and startling that it may completely revise our conception of heart disease. . . . Dr. Sandler does not believe that the fat content of the diet is responsible for the recent increase of heart disease. This sounds incredible, based on a huge amount of research that has been done on cholesterol and fat, but perhaps eventually it will be found

[85]

that Dr. Sandler's low carbohydrate diet will be more effective in curing heart disease than the low fat diet."

We went on to point out that doctors were stressing the fat-heart disease relationship and ignoring other significant factors such as exercise and the consumption of other types of foods. "They also ignore the over-consumption of sugar in the United States, which was 103 pounds per year per person in 1940, whereas in Italy (relatively low in heart disease) it was only 21 pounds. It is probably a combination of three factors— low sugar consumption, low fat consumption and increased exercise in Italy which keeps their heart disease rate down."

Dr. Sandler described many cases in which the low-carbohydrate diet he devised had been successful in giving relief from attacks of heart pain, and preventing their recurrence. One of the clues that convinced Dr. Sandler of the dangers of carbohydrates and sugar to heart cases was the fact that in diabetics, heart disease is more serious, occurs at an earlier age and is more common.

Dr. Sandler said then, that he was not convinced that hardening of the arteries is necessarily a reliable indicator of heart attack. "Many victims of heart attacks, especially those between 20 and 40 years, show no evidence of arteriosclerosis at necropsy (autopsy)."

Dr. Sandler bravely took on the cholesterol controversy and pointed out that researchers have overlooked the fact that the body can make cholesterol from sugar and starch as well as from fat. He insisted, however, that cholesterol really has nothing to do with heart at-

[86]

tack caused by arteriosclerosis, because many persons with arteriosclerosis do not show elevation of the blood cholesterol.

Another argument against the fatty theory, according to Dr. Sandler, is the fact that "the Eskimo living within the Arctic Circle is notoriously free of arteriosclerosis and heart attacks and yet consumes an extremely high-fat diet compared with the average diet of Americans in the United States. The Eskimo lives entirely on protein and fat in the form of meat, fish and blubber."

As far back as 1937 Dr. Sandler was making sugar tests of the blood in his patients, and in more than half of them he saw evidence of low blood sugar due to high carbohydrate intake. The heart muscle requires a steady supply of sugar (glucose) in order to function normally. If there isn't enough, this muscle stops working at peak efficiency and death eventually ensues. To quote Dr. Sandler, "I also wish to emphasize the fact that the blood sugar supply to the central nervous system is particularly important, because abnormal fluctuations in the blood sugar level affect not only the function of the heart but also the function of the central nervous system. Many of the symptoms experienced by heart patients are due directly to the effects of the fall in blood sugar on the cells of the brain and the spinal cord. The blood sugar must not only be supplied continuously, but must also be maintained at optimum level, 80 milligrams per 100 cc. When the blood sugar falls below 80 milligrams certain organs, especially the central nervous system, would be embarrassed and

[87]

signs and symptoms of disturbance in the function make their appearance. The severity of the signs and symptoms will depend on how low and at what rate the blood sugar falls."

In Sandler's opinion pressure chest pains of angina in a heart condition are caused by rapid and sharp fall in blood sugar level. He claims to have cured many such conditions by a diet capable of preventing the abnormal fluctuations in blood sugar levels. The diet is said to be effective in all age groups. Dr. Sandler explains the effect of sugar on the heart's action in this way: "Heart muscle is made up of innumerable muscle cells. Like all muscle tissue, it needs certain nutrients to perform its work of contraction and relaxation. The chief nutrients are sugar and oxygen, both of which are brought to the muscle by the blood . . . Any significant interference with the supply of sugar or oxygen will embarrass heart action, and the degree of interference will determine the degree of embarrassment— from a mild fleeting chest pain to the severe crushing pain of the fatal heart attack."

It is the violent fluctuations in the blood sugar that create the most trouble, says Dr. Sandler. Eating a meal rich in carbohydrates will do that because first it raises the blood sugar, then lowers it. "The rapid rate of change in the downward direction results in a severe environmental change for the heart muscle, to which it fails to accommodate readily and so the muscle is embarrassed and the symptoms of pain are felt by the patient." Nicotine and caffeine cause a rise in the blood sugar. That's why, when blood sugar is low between meals, a pick-me-up cigarette or cup of coffee seems to help. This raises the blood sugar and contributes to the violent fluctuations that Sandler warned against.

In addition to sugar, oxygen is important to the helpful operation of the heart muscle. "It has been shown that a cell utilizes oxygen in proportion as it utilizes sugar. But oxygen is useful to the cell only if there is some fuel to burn (oxidize) for the production of energy. The blood may be normally saturated with oxygen but if the blood sugar level is half what it should be, the body will consume less than normal oxygen . . . It has been accepted by many that the immediate cause of heart pain is an acute oxygen lack on the part of the heart muscle." Of course vitamin E is a conserver of oxygen in the body and therefore, together with a high protein diet and plenty of exercise, works well to prevent heart attack.

Dr. Sandler recommends that the following foods should be avoided: sugar, soft drinks, ice cream, ices, sherbets, cakes, candies, cookies, wafers, pastries, pies, fruit juices, canned and preserved foods, jams, jellies, marmalades, puddings, custards and syrups. He recommended that high starch foods such as beans, corn, cereals of all kinds be eaten in reduced quantity. There are many specific recommendations in the book, but basically the Sandler diet is high protein (plenty of animal foods) and low carbohydrate.

[89]

Part Four:

VITAMINS THAT BENEFIT THE HEART

CHAPTER X

The Role of Vitamin C

What is often taken for heart disease on the reading of an abnormal electrocardiogram tracing, may actually be a deficiency of vitamin C, J. Shafar, M.D. suggests in *The Lancet* (July 22, 1967). He reports on two patients suffering from scurvy whose electrocardiograms gave every indication of heart trouble. After a week on supplementary vitamin C, the patients' readings reverted to normal.

According to Dr. Shafar this situation is more common than most clinicians realize, especially where older persons are concerned. Subclinical deficiencies of vitamin C occur frequently in the elderly because of a general prevalence of malnutrition in this age group. Many have particular food fetishes or suffer from digestive diseases which lead them to avoid fresh, uncooked vitamin C-rich foods. Sometimes doctors are to blame: "I have used the term 'iatrogenic scurvy' for those cases where scurvy arises from restrictions of diet accepted on medical evidence and where the ill effects of the absence of the prohibited foods are not offset by vitamin supplementation," says Shafar.

The link between circulatory troubles and a shortage of vitamin C is not new. Some years ago Dr. J. C. Paterson, a pathologist, reported in the *Canadian Medical Association Journal* that he frequently found capillary hemorrhages at the very location of a fatal blood clot. He began to relate this type of capillary damage to coronary thrombosis. Paterson's conclusion is supported by Ziegler's classic, *General Pathology,* eighth edition, which lists changes in the blood vessel wall as one of the three major causes of thrombosis. When any kind of a breakdown occurs in such circulatory tissues, experienced pathologists have learned to suspect a shortage of vitamin C.

The cells that form the artery walls like all other cells are held together by collagen, sometimes called "the cement of life." Normally this intercellular cement maintains a firmness like a well-set gel. When vitamin C is deficient, this "glue" between the cell walls becomes watery and seeps into the bloodstream. Biochemists can spot a vitamin C deficiency by examining the blood for increased serum-glycoprotein, one of the main constituents of the loosened collagen. It is revealing that a high glycoprotein reading is present in a number of disease conditions including rheumatic diseases, colds, infections, cancer and myocardial infarction, a serious heart disorder. As expected, a definite

[94]

deficiency of vitamin C (the key to glycoprotein release) is found in these same conditions, all named as
frequent forerunners of thrombosis. (*Proceedings of the
Staff Meetings at the Mayo Clinic,* 31: 1956, points
out the striking concurrence of cancer and thrombosis.)

Dr. Paterson found evidence to back up his conclusion about the connection between vitamin C deficiency and coronary thrombosis in hospital records.
They showed that 81 per cent of coronary cases in
hospitals have a subnormal blood plasma level of vitamin C, compared with 55.8 per cent of a similar non-
coronary group.

G. C. Willis in *The Report of the Annual Meeting
and Proceedings of the Royal College of Physicians
and Surgeons of Canada* (October 30-31, 1953) said
that scurvy, an extreme deficiency of vitamin C, is effective in producing damage to the arteries of experimental guinea pigs, identical to that seen in the human
disease. In other studies of blood vessels, doctors found
fatty deposits in the capillaries and small veins of experimental animals as well as humans when vitamin C
was in short supply. Finally, widespread arteriosclerosis
and thrombosis in young people who died of malnutrition in prison camps of World War II was reported
by French researchers. It is reasonable to assume that
they suffered from a lack of vitamin C. Certainly they
were not the victims of cholesterol overfeeding.

A major new therapeutic role for ascorbic acid came
to light recently as a result of research studies on animals carried out by Dr. Richard Bing of Wayne State
University in Detroit, who has found it to be of great

[95]

value in promoting healing after myocardial infarction, a life-threatening stage of coronary disease.

Because heart failure causes not only vascular incapacity and restriction of capillary blood flow, but also changes in enzyme patterns, Dr. Bing did enzyme studies which showed that the process of repair in the damaged heart muscle can be accelerated by three different treatments: ascorbic acid, the anabolic steroids and a new treatment called the Sodi-Pallares polarizing therapy.

Dr. Demetrio Sodi-Pallares of the National Institute of Cardiology in Mexico used the term 'polarizing therapy' to refer to an electrolyte therapy utilizing a combination of diet and solution of glucose, insulin, and potassium chloride which contributes to repolarization (the orderly arrangement of nuclei and tissue permitting normal life activities, such as cell regeneration and rhythmic contraction and expansion) of myocardial fibers, the first step in the restoration of heart health. Dr. Sodi-Pallares told a meeting of the New York Academy of Sciences in January, 1967 that "digitalis compounds and diuretic drugs in heart failure, the vasodilator agents in angina and coronary insufficiency, the hypotensive drugs and diuretics in hypertension, have yielded their place of honor to this treatment."

Vitamin Avoids Drug Dangers

Supplementing the work of Dr. Sodi-Pallares, Dr. Bing of Detroit achieved the effect of the 'polarizing therapy' using ascorbic acid which plays a vital role in cellular metabolism. The insulin in the original polar-

[96]

izing solution, Dr. Bing told *Prevention,* acts like a growth hormone, stimulating the growth of new tissue. But insulin can promote dangerous complications, especially where there is diabetes or problems of renal function. Potassium is a valuable adjunct in this therapy because it helps restore the alkaline balance necessary for optimal regularity of the heart beat. Severe heart attack is usually accompanied by severe acidosis. But potassium intake, too, must be carefully regulated. Over-dosage can produce weakness, confusion, paresthesia, and an irregular heartbeat.

Use of the anabolic steroids, while helpful in providing the adrenal hormone which triggers heart action and promotes the growth of new cells, is riddled with dangerous side-effects. Continued use of cortisone, for instance, tends to deplete the system of calcium, another element vital to the health of the heart. Patients on cortisone develop abnormally round faces and abnormal growths of hair. Steroids can also cause ulcers, high blood pressure and diabetes.

Of the three therapies found effective in promoting the regeneration of the heart muscle, the only one without any deleterious side-effects is vitamin C.

This is a dramatic new role for ascorbic acid. But it is not surprising. What a vitamin helps to prevent, it often helps to cure and the effect of vitamin C on cardiovascular health is well known.

CHAPTER XI

B Vitamins and Sugar

The practice of eating refined white sugar results in robbing the body of its vitamin B. It is that portion of vitamin B called thiamin which is destroyed. Thiamin is one of the most important vitamins for good health. It is necessary for growth, good appetite and smooth functioning of the digestive tract. It plays so big a part in nerve health that it is called the "morale" vitamin. Most important of all, thiamin is vitally concerned with the digestion and assimilation of all carbohydrate foods —the sugars and starches. It must be present in considerable quantity if these foods are to be used at all by the body.

Thiamin is stolen from our bodies by these robber foods—white sugar, synthetic sugar, white flour, prepared cereals and many other refined and processed foods. If you eat carbohydrates in natural forms you do not experience any thiamin deficiency because the thiamin to digest the sugar or starch is present in the natural food. For instance, blackstrap molasses contains a great deal of natural sugar. It also has thiamin and a number of the other B vitamins, ready to go to work. Refined white sugar is the product that remains after all these B vitamins as well as many other valuable minerals have been removed from the molasses. When you eat white sugar in coffee, cakes, candies, pies, ice cream and soft drinks, you are presenting your digestive tract with large quantities of sugar to be digested and no thiamin or other B vitamins to aid in the process. In order to handle this sugar at all, the body must steal thiamin from other processes and from its storage places in the liver, kidney and heart. This means that if you eat much white sugar, if you eat some of it every day, you are almost bound to suffer from thiamin deficiency. If you are a heart case such dietary habit is cold suicide as you shall soon see. We might express it thus: Sugar equals vitamin B deficiency equals heart trouble.

Now let us proceed into a discussion of the medical writings which show the relationship between heart trouble and vitamin B deficiency. In a book called *The Avitaminoses* by Walter H. Eddy, Ph.D., and Gilbert Dalldorf, M.D. (published by The Williams & Wilkins Company), appears the statement, "Thiamin deficiency impairs the function of the heart, increases the tendency to extravascular fluid collections and results in terminal cardiac standstill." The authors show how the famous English research physician, Sir Robert McCar-

[99]

rison, in experiments with pigeons, produced cardiac (heart) changes in them by feeding them a vitamin B deficient diet. Eddy and Dalldorf describe another experiment in which congestive heart failure was produced in pigeons and then cured by thiamin.

In the book *Nutrition and Diet in Health and Disease* by James S. McLester, M.D. (W. B. Saunders Company), it is stated that a thiamin deficiency causes a degeneration in the heart muscles. Pigs that were fed a thiamin-free diet showed a scarring in the right side of the heart.

E. V. McCollum, Ph.D., Sc.D., L.L.D., in *The Newer Knowledge of Nutrition* (The Macmillan Company), shows that the normal heart rate of the rat is 500 to 550 beats per minute but when they are fed a diet low in thiamin for about three weeks the rate goes down to about 350 per minute. In fact this reduction is so dependable an occurrence on lowering the thiamin intake that it is used in laboratories to test the thiamin content of certain vitamin products. McCollum states that where the heart rate of deficient animals went down, it could be brought up again automatically within four hours after the administration of thiamin.

In the book *Vitaminology* by Walter H. Eddy, M.D., (Williams and Wilkins), the fact is discussed that a thiamin deficiency leads to beriberi disease. He says, "A definite relation of thiamin deficiency to cardiac (heart) function has long been recognized. . . . The characteristics of beriberi heart in human subjects are enlargement (usually of the right side), decreased circulation time, elevated or normal venous pressure, less

[100]

difference than normal between the oxygen content of arterial and venous blood, and usually rapid recovery following thiamin therapy. Similar effects are observed in patients developing thiamin deficiency through the excessive use of alcohol. In both these cases the heart is tremendously dilated and the edema (swelling) is massive." This book is just chock full of instances of heart damage where the thiamin in the diet is lowered, but there is one statement which is extremely significant: "The effect of thiamin was interpreted as increasing arterial tone."

In the *New Zealand Medical Journal* for June, 1952, there is an article by G. L. Brinkman, M.D., in which four unfamiliar forms of heart failure are described due to faulty nutrition, mostly a lack of thiamin.

There are other parts of vitamin B complex which should also be considered in the treatment of this subject. For example—biotin. A deficiency of biotin produces symptoms of lassitude, sleepiness, muscular pains, loss of appetite, pallor, dryness of skin, disturbances of the nervous system and a feeling of distress in the region of the heart.

In our discussion of vitamin C, we showed how it is a factor in fortifying the body against conditions of stress. There seems to be evidence also that vitamin B serves the same purpose. The B fractions which are so involved include pantothenic acid, riboflavin, folic acid and vitamin B_{12} as well as our old friend thiamin. The particular site of trouble caused by their deficiencies which reduces ability to withstand stress is in the adrenal glands.

[101]

In one case an investigator by the name of Rolli found that rats who were on a diet deficient in pantothenic acid showed an inability of the white blood cells to withstand stress. There is a considerable amount of animal experimental data which proves conclusively that both vitamin B and vitamin C factors enable the body to withstand tension-caused illness.

The consumption of sugar and alcohol rob the body of vitamin B. There are other practices that do the same thing. White flour, prepared cereals and many other refined foods are serious offenders in this regard, because the vitamin B has been removed, but it is badly needed to aid the digestion of carbohydrates.

Sleeping pills should not be taken, for the same reason. The barbiturates block the progress of carbohydrate metabolism and so add to the difficulty of securing enough thiamin.

Estrogen, a hormone administered in certain diseases, especially where individuals are inclined to be deficient in the B vitamins will greatly cut down three of the B complexes—thiamin, riboflavin and niacin.

The sulfa drugs are mentioned in all literature dealing with vitamin enemies. Some of the B vitamins are manufactured in our intestines, so that, even if our diet is lacking in B vitamins, we may still get by, so long as the friendly "intestinal flora" go on producing B vitamins for us. The sulfa drugs upset this whole machinery and, if given long enough, they cut off this supply of vitamins. This is why pneumonia patients, for instance, whose doctors give them large doses of sulfa drugs, may recover almost miraculously from the disease, but find

[102]

that they are left in a state of terrible depression, fatigue and digestive disorder which may go on for years until they catch up on the necessary supply of B vitamins.

We can see, therefore, that if we assure ourselves sufficient vitamin B, preferably in the form of supplements to the regular diet, such as brewer's yeast, desiccated liver, wheat germ and blackstrap molasses, we will be moving in the right direction towards preventing an undue accumulation of fatty deposits in the artery walls.

CHAPTER XII

Thiamin

A very convincing demonstration of the relationship between carbohydrate consumption, thiamin shortage and incipient heart trouble among relatively healthy individuals appears in *The International Journal for Vitamin Research* (37, No. 4, 1967) by E. Cheraskin, M.D., D.M.D., professor and chairman of the Department of Oral Medicine at the University of Alabama Medical Center, and associates. Cheraskin recruited 74 dentists and their wives to answer the questions in the standard Cornell Medical Index Health Questionnaire dealing with cardiovascular symptoms and signs: ("Do you have pains in the heart or the chest?" "Are you often bothered by thumping of the heart?" "Does heart trouble run in your family?" "Do you get out of breath long before anyone else?" etc.) Twenty-six of the men and 15 of the women (a total of 55.4 per cent) had no cardiovascular complaints whatsoever, but 16 per cent of the total group had at least one complaint, and 10.8 per cent had two complaints. One woman said yes to 7 out of 13 questions that might indicate cardiovascular problems.

The same group participated in a 7-day dietary survey through which the researchers calculated the daily thiamin intake. The subjects with the most heart problems, it turned out, were the older people in the study who consumed the least thiamin.

In order to compare the cardiovascular complaints to dietary consumption, the dentists and their wives were divided into two equal sub-groups: of these 74 individuals, 37 consumed .13 to .91 milligrams of thiamin a day (Group 1); the remaining 37 consumed .92 to 2.95 milligrams of thiamin a day (Group 2). The same division was done for consumption of non-processed carbohydrates and processed carbohydrates.

When all of these groups were compared, the two groups with the highest number of cardiovascular complaints were also found to have a higher consumption of processed carbohydrates and a lower consumption of thiamin than the rest. "Additionally," says Cheraskin, "the three groups with the highest mean cardiovascular scores (the most complaints) have a common denominator of smaller thiamin consumption." In other words, the paper was able to demonstrate that persons with heart complaints tend to be those who consume more carbohydrates and less thiamin. (It is important to note that, when carbohydrates are consumed, increased amounts of thiamin are necessary to process them in the system.) "It should be underlined that the relationships observed here do not, in themselves, prove cause-and-effect. However, it is noteworthy that the findings are consistent with other reports indicating the relationship of carbohydrate consumption to cardiovascular disease."

Although Dr. Cheraskin is among the most renowned and influential of the research scientists who have delved into the problem of carbohydrates, thiamin and heart disease, he properly calls attention to the many previous experiments that support this relationship. The major differences between Cheraskin's work and that of other scientists is that his attempts have included living humans. Others have worked largely with laboratory animals or deceased humans.

Earl E. Aldinger, Ph.D., from the Department of Medicine, Tulane School of Medicine, put living rats on a thiamin-free diet for 5 weeks. During that time the tissues surrounding the heart showed a marked loss (69 per cent) of tension and elasticity. The animals were also inclined toward an erratic heartbeat. As the weeks without thiamin went on, the irregularity was more and more pronounced. Many of the rats died during the experiment.

The role of thiamin in heart failure was touched on briefly in *Nutrition Reviews* (October, 1955). M. G. Wohl, *et al.* did their testing on human cadavers. Wohl measured the thiamin content of the heart muscle and of the liver and kidney tissues in 12 patients who died from heart failure with evidence of various kinds of severe organic heart disease.

These tissues were compared with similar tissues

[106]

taken from 10 patients who had no heart disease and who died of other causes. The doctors found a consistent decrease in the average thiamin content of the heart muscle in the cardiac patients as compared with the control subjects.

The total thiamin in the "noncardiacs" was 1.37 micrograms per gram of tissue as compared to .60 micrograms for the cardiac subjects. *Nutrition Reviews* commented, "Because of the nature of the study it was presumably impossible for the author to obtain histories of food intake on either the cardiacs or control individuals prior to death so that these could be compared. The assumption would seem valid that the patients dying of severe cardiac disease had not been well nourished for a considerable period of time prior to death. Whether the deficiencies found were sufficient to impair the metabolism of heart muscle was not known, although as the authors indicate, these evidences of under-nutrition with respect to thiamin are certainly suggested."

[107]

CHAPTER XIII

Vitamin B₁₅ Helps the Heart

Up to now, practically nothing has been known about vitamin B₁₅ and its role, if any, in human metabolism. The latest edition of the *Merck Index,* an authoritative encyclopedia for pharmacists, chemists, and doctors, merely describes the chemistry of this vitamin, but has nothing to suggest as to what it may be useful for. In fact, pangamic acid (B₁₅) has been called a vitamin only by virtue of its having been discovered in certain foods that are sources of the B complex vitamins— notably, brewer's yeast and seeds.

Pangamic acid is one of those substances that the "nutritional authorities" of the Food and Drug Administration consider of no value in human nutrition, because they don't know of any such value, and they like to think that what they know about nutrition is all that there is to know and all that will ever be known.

[108]

This arrogant attitude, of course, is the reverse of that of many nutritional authorities like J. I. Rodale, who have faith in the wisdom of nature and know that a substance like pangamic acid, non-toxic and part of the B complex of vitamins, must have a purpose even if it is not yet discovered.

This, of course, is one of the basic reasons why *Prevention* has always recommended vitamin supplements, like brewer's yeast, made of the whole foods that contain the vitamins, as superior to purified vitamin substances. That our point of view is the correct one and the necessary one for any person interested in peak health, is once more borne out by a Russian research study published in *Reports of the Academy of Sciences, U.S.S.R.* (144, 3, 1962).

Retards Asphyxiation

It is only a preliminary report that has been published so far, yet it was able to arrive at the definite conclusion that "our results indicate that vitamin B15 increases general and myocardial resistance to hypoxia." Coming from a team of prominent Russian scientists (Dokukin, Konstantinova, Chechulin, and Bukin), this conclusion is in itself important, and opens a door to further investigations that might be of prime significance.

Hypoxia simply means an insufficient supply of oxygen to living tissue. The myocardium is the muscle tissue of the heart, tissue that makes a continual, strong demand for oxygen and that quickly fails when the

[109]

oxygen supply is inadequate. There are many reasons why, at any given time, the heart and other tissues might not receive enough oxygen. There might be an anemic condition of the blood, causing hypoxia at a time of unusual physical effort such as unaccustomed running or shoveling snow. There is sometimes difficulty in starting the breathing of a newborn baby, and until the breathing actually begins, there is hypoxia. Carbon monoxide poisoning—almost a chronic condition in the polluted air of large cities— will induce hypoxia. Failure or weakness of the respiratory system, whether temporary or chronic, will have the same result. It is not a problem that occurs for everyone, but it occurs enough times for people so that any substance that increases our ability to survive such a crisis becomes an important substance for that reason alone.

That, it seems, is just what pangamic acid does for us.

Experimental Proof

The Russian scientists carried out their experiments on large numbers of mice, rats, cats, and dogs. The animals were given dosages of vitamin B$_{15}$ in amounts of from 150 to 500 milligrams for each kilogram of weight. Then the animals were placed in sealed containers and the process of gradual asphyxiation was observed.

(Though the knowledge gained from these experiments was important, we do not condone the cruelty that was involved in the experiments themselves. It seems to us that scientists capable of conducting bril-

[110]

liant experiments could well apply some of their brilliance to devising more humane methods.)

Twenty minutes after the start of the experiment, it was found that 9 per cent of the control (no pangamic acid) animals had died, as compared with only 3.3 per cent of the animals that had been fortified with the vitamin.

The Russian scientific team offered a persuasive explanation of why this should be so. The direct action of pangamic acid, they say, is to stimulate the hypophysis of the supra-renal glands. These are glands located in the body just above the kidneys, hence the name. The hypophysis is a kind of bump on each, which the Russian investigators state has an important detoxifying function. By stimulating this activity, they believe, pangamic acid retards the accumulation of toxic waste that results from an insufficiency of oxygen. Thus the hypoxia does less damage, and a longer period of time remains for normal oxygen metabolism to be reestablished without fundamental damage to the organism.

The Russians offered this preliminary report to urge the use of pangamic acid as a drug in heart surgery, when for a time the flow of blood to the heart must be cut off and hypoxia results. Certainly it should be of value for this purpose.

How about vitamin B15 in nutrition, however? In Russia, that cannot represent any great problem. Sunflower seeds are eaten in large quantity by practically everyone. These seeds contain a rich supply of vitamin B15, and we may assume that most Russians get a suf-

[111]

ficiency of the vitamin in this way. Improved ability to endure the oxygen-depletion of heavy exercise could well be a partial explanation for the superior stamina and physical condition of young Russians, as compared to young Americans, a matter that has received a great deal of comment lately.

Unlike Russians, most Americans don't eat either seeds or brewer's yeast for fear of being considered food faddists and health nuts. We can assume, therefore, that the American diet is generally deficient in this vitamin. It is not even included in most vitamin supplements, unless they are natural supplements. Its dietary sources are very few, indeed. Aside from seeds and brewer's yeast, the vitamin is found also in horse liver, ox blood, and rice bran. None of these is exactly a staple on the American table.

We must, therefore, assume that most Americans get little or no pangamic acid. This means that Americans have less ability to survive temporary conditions of oxygen insufficiency. The inevitable result would seem to be a larger number of heart attacks and less ability to recover from such attacks. Can this be the reason, or one of the reasons, why the rate of cardiac deaths in the United States is sharply on the increase?

Here is a field wide open for investigation. Without irrefutable scientific evidence, we cannot say that it is so. But it seems a reasonable conclusion from the facts that have already been scientifically demonstrated. Having learned these facts, we urge our readers to protect themselves with a good intake of pangamic acid.

You may be sure that in the sunflower and pumpkin

seeds and in the brewer's yeast, you will also be getting other protective factors that have not yet been dis- covered or whose values are still unknown, but which will go ahead and work for you regardless of whether or not they have been sanctioned by the Committee on Nutrition of the AMA.

CHAPTER XIV

How Vitamins Cope
with Cholesterol

If the mountains of publicity have you worried about the cholesterol level in your own body, you will be relieved to know that scientists have shown that a diet high in nutrients is probably your best defense against a cholesterol problem. Eating properly and getting the proper amount of exercise is better, say the scientists, than any new drug, crash diet or anything else that's been developed to cash in on the cholesterol phobia that has gripped the United States. Proper cholesterol levels are achieved experimentally in high cholesterol patients by the use of various nutrients added to a stock diet. If your regular diet is planned to include such nutrients as a matter of course, you can rest easy about the likelihood of a cholesterol pile-up. Nutrients

[114]

help the body to work smoothly. A body working as it should can make proper use of the cholesterol it needs and eliminate the rest naturally.

Experimenters have seemed surprised at the success they had in controlling levels with simple nutrients. We would have been surprised at any other result. Our instinct is always to look to the use of proper diet and natural food supplements to handle effectively any problem which, like cholesterol accumulation, is essentially one of metabolism.

Most prominent, in the experimental efforts to use a nutrient in controlling the amount of cholesterol in the blood stream, has been niacin, one of the B complex fractions. Suspicions of this relationship show up in our files as far back as 1956. *Scope Weekly* (August 15, 1956) told of work done at the Mayo Clinic, resulting in favorable findings in 9 out of 13 patients observed for 12 weeks, during which time they were given large daily doses of niacin (nicotinic acid). Even over the relatively short period of 4 weeks, niacin (3 grams per day) was shown to lower cholesterol in the blood stream in 3 out of 5 cases. In cases where cholesterol levels failed to respond, dosage was upped to 4 to 6 grams daily.

In 1957 the Bakery Foods Foundation of Canada reported similarly in *Nutrition Views and News* (Summer Issue). Both rabbits and humans were tested, and both were positively affected by niacin with a lowering of cholesterol.

A 2-year study by a group of Saskatchewan scientists on niacin and its effect on cholesterol, appearing in the

[115]

Canadian Medical Association Journal (December 15, 1957), secured the relationship once and for all. Corroborative reports came in *Circulation* (17: 497, 1958) and the *Canadian Medical Association Journal* (78: 402, 1958) reinforcing the principle. In the *British Medical Journal* (September 20, 1958), Altschul and Hoffer wrote: "It seems well-established that nicotinic acid in relatively high doses decreases serum cholesterol in healthy and sick human beings."

It took a long time for the news about niacin's value as an anti-cholesterol agent to filter through to the nation's popular news media. However, *Newsweek* did publish in the November 9, 1959 issue a small note which named the B vitamin as "the most effective way to reduce blood cholesterol levels."

Interesting to observe, there is still considerable puzzlement in medical minds as to why niacin would have such an effect on the cholesterol level. Also puzzling to most researchers is the mild, but definite, reaction suffered by many patients given niacin in large amounts. In general, flushing of the skin, and dilation of the blood vessels commonly occur. Some researchers saw irritation of the intestinal tract and liver malfunction resulting as well. The workers all seemed to agree that niacin given at these high levels no longer operates as a vitamin, but rather as a drug. "It has been noted that the nicotinic acid (niacin) will produce vasodilation and pruritus (iching) when administered at this level, changes which are not noted when it is administered at vitamin levels."

It is apparent from the research that has been done

[116]

with niacin that it has a definite value in achieving the proper cholesterol balance in the body. However, we are sure that this balance was meant by Nature to be *maintained* rather than achieved. If large doses of niacin used therapeutically will restore a proper cholesterol reading, then we believe that regular intake of niacin as part of a diet rich in the B complex, as it occurs in brewer's yeast, desiccated liver and wheat germ, would never have let the cholesterol rise to a dangerous accumulation in the first place.

While niacin might be the most widely recognized and accepted treatment in general medicine for lowering cholesterol, researchers have become excited about other nutrients in this connection. In the *Medical Journal of Australia* (2: 307, 1961) vitamins A and D were described as successfully-employed tools in fighting high cholesterol levels in humans. The period of observation covered 5½ years and included 136 patients, with 271 other patients serving as controls. In the group to whom vitamins A and D were given, coronary heart disease developed in only 5.8 per cent, as opposed to its development in 15.8 per cent of those not treated—a 3-fold increase in incidence because the control group didn't receive the A and D supplementation!

It was shown in this report that the vitamins were most effective in reducing the high level cholesterol as opposed to the lower (though above normal) levels: "Following the administration of vitamins A and D, there was a highly significant reduction of the mean serum cholesterol level in 13 men with an initial level

[117]

of 250 milligrams per milliliter or more, but there were no significant changes of cholesterol in those with smaller initial levels." This means to us that the body is ready to take correction when it is necessary by making use of supplementary nutrients; when levels are safe enough, such help is unnecessary and, therefore, rejected. However, vitamin A is now known to be necessary to cholesterol processing. The authors concluded: "There is evidence that vitamin A deficiency impairs cholesterol metabolism, that supplements of this vitamin reduce hypercholesterolemia (high cholesterol), and possibly can reverse atheroma."

R. R. Becker and associates reported in the *Journal of the American Chemical Society*, volume 75, page 2020, 1953, on the value of ascorbic acid, or vitamin C, in the proper use of cholesterol by the body. Their study was conducted on guinea pigs. The guinea pigs were divided into three groups. The first group was given a normal ration and was allowed to eat at will. The cholesterol reading for this group of guinea pigs ranged from 80 to 100. A second group was deprived of some vitamin C—enough to produce a mild form of scurvy. This group showed readings of 170. Where severe scurvy was induced by the deprivation of vitamin C for from 3 to 4 weeks, readings of cholesterol went up to 600.

The material showed that vitamin C is essential in helping the body to process cholesterol so that it does not pile up in the system and create problems for the circulation.

The important part played by vitamin E in the control of cholesterol levels is suggested by a letter to *The Lancet* (April 18, 1962). As we know, one of the important services vitamin E performs is retention of oxygen in the blood stream. The authors attributed to a shortage of oxygen interference with certain enzyme action, which leads to improper synthesis of phospholipids and protein. Both of these, in turn, are important in the transportation and the dispersion of cholesterol and other lipids. This restricted movement of cholesterol allows for its accumulation on the inner part of the arterial wall.

Inclusion of supplemental vitamin E in the diet would act to maintain a desirable oxygen level in the blood. The oxygen would then act in its proper role as assistant in this one enzyme function: to encourage proper distribution of cholesterol in the blood stream.

The obvious conclusion to be drawn from all of this material, showing that the specific elements contained in natural food have a healthful effect on serum cholesterol levels, is simply that such food, if properly scheduled in the regular diet, plus exercise, will help the average person to maintain a cholesterol level which is proper to his size and weight.

We would much prefer to see the individual include brewer's yeast, wheat germ and the organ meats in his regular daily ration, rather than to concentrate on large amounts of a specific B vitamin as a therapeutic measure to lower cholesterol. We would prefer him to eat fresh fruits and vegetables for a proper vitamin C intake as well as a good supply of pectin, rather than have him wait for the day when his serum cholesterol

[119]

is so high that he must take injections of vitamin C in order to normalize it.

We believe that it is not the amount of cholesterol which one takes but the body's readiness to handle cholesterol as it should that is important. A normal healthy body is bound to have a normal healthy cholesterol level.

Vitamin C and Cholesterol

There are several researches performed in the last few years which prove that vitamin C is an important factor in keeping down the cholesterol in the blood. One of the most remarkable of them has come out of Russia and was written up in *Terapevtichevski Archiv.* vol. 28, page 59, 1956. (The translation was done by Julius Nemetz of Allentown, Pennsylvania.) This article proves that vitamin C is both a preventive and a cure of atherosclerosis. According to it, Dr. I. A. Miasnikov was able to prove that within a few hours after administering vitamin C (ascorbic acid) her patients showed a sharp decline in the cholesterol level of the blood. In 1952 she proved graphically that vitamin C could stop artificially induced atherosclerosis. These observations were confirmed by co-workers L. A. Tiapinoi, G. N. Loubman and E. M. Berkoviskin.

In 1949 Dr. Miasnikov began the study of patients suffering from hypertension (high blood pressure) and atherosclerosis. These patients had been treated with the usual hygienic methods, such as periods of rest and work, physical exercise, elimination of excess fats and alcoholic beverages. Different medications were also

[120]

given them, with apparently little change in their condition. But in the last two years she began to give them vitamin C.

Here is part of Dr. Miasnikov's report regarding the effect of this vitamin. First, the amount of cholesterol in the blood was checked, before administering the vitamin C, and then the amount of cholesterol was determined after the 1st, 2nd, 3rd and 4th hours, after giving the patients ½ gram of ascorbic acid (vitamin C). Of the 35 patients, 28 had an excess of cholesterol and 7 had between 150 and 180 mgs. of cholesterol. In those 7 patients whose cholesterol was normal, the use of ascorbic acid did not change the level of cholesterol. But in those with high cholesterol, the level was lowered considerably. In 15 patients the percentage of cholesterol came down 15 per cent. In 8 patients it came down 16 to 30 per cent; in 5 patients 31 to 50 per cent. A definite sharp decline of cholesterol in the blood was noted within a 24-hour period after the use of ascorbic acid, and a normalizing effect by the end of the experimental period.

The following methods were pursued: When the patient was admitted to the hospital, tests were taken every three hours and .5 grams of ascorbic acid (500 milligrams) were given twice daily. The patient was given a low-fat diet and was told to try to keep calm emotionally, to abstain from alcoholic beverages and to do a little physical work. Within a period of from 10 to 30 days the cholesterol became normal in most cases. After completing this course of treatments, the patients would come a few times a year for a .5 gram

[121]

injection of ascorbic acid. In our opinion, the taking of a natural vitamin C product would be even more effective.

Usually these patients would complain of headaches, noises in the head, dizziness, loss of memory, lowered working ability, sharp disturbances of sleep, and lowered ability to hear and see.

Ascorbic acid (vitamin C) was used in curing 106 patients who had atherosclerosis. Of these patients, only 7 had cholesterol under 180. In 23 the amount was between 180 and 200. 45 had 201 to 250, 16 patients 251 to 300, 7 had 301 to 350, 5 had 351 to 400, and 3 cases had over 400 mg. After the first course of treatments, 92 patients showed a sharp decline of cholesterol in the blood, 3 patients declined 50 per cent, 10 patients 41 per cent to 50 per cent, 13 patients declined 31 to 40 per cent, 25 patients 21 to 30 per cent, 30 patients 11 to 20 per cent, and 11 patients 10 per cent. In 11 cases where the reading was 200 there was scarcely any change. The improved conditions became noticeable after the first few days of the treatments. Headaches and noises in the head disappeared, memory improved and sleep became sound.

Here is a description of a typical case: Patient A was kept on non-vitamin medications from 1951 to 1954 without any improvement. He was suffering with headaches, noises in the head, pain around the heart extending to the entire left arm. He also could not sleep more than 3 to 4 hours a night. He was irritable and had tremors in the fingers and eyelids. His pulse was 68 and the tone of the heart beats was dull (hard

[122]

to hear). Analysis of blood and urine was normal, but cholesterol was high (400). The patient was given 1000 milligrams (1 gram) of ascorbic acid daily for 30 days, upon which the cholesterol came down to 180. After 10 days of treatment he began to feel fine and was able to work a little, which he could not do before. Three months later he kept on feeling well and the cholesterol remained at between 160 and 190.

Another case: Patient K, born in 1882, was under observation since the fall of 1949. In June, 1952 her atherosclerosis was beginning to get worse. In July, 1952 the patient went through a severe emotional experience and she developed a 240/140 blood pressure, which was extremely high. She was treated with the usual bromides and other medications, was made to feel comfortable and her blood pressure came down to 170/100. However, insignificant emotional upsets would drive her blood pressure up to 220/110 and 260/140. By September, 1955 it was very hard to live with her. She was irritable, had headaches; loss of memory, and could not sleep more than 3 to 4 hours a night. Her heart beats were dull. She had tremors in her fingers and eyelids and suffered from a general weakened condition. Her heart became enlarged, pulse weak, cholesterol 320.

Ascorbic acid was given her in large doses, and on the second day, the cholesterol came down to normal. Her condition improved, and most of the unpleasant symptoms disappeared. After 9 days of the treatments, the blood pressure came down to normal.

In summary the article says: (1) The literature and

[123]

our observations indicate that ascorbic acid normalizes the level of cholesterol in the blood. From the first dose of $\frac{1}{2}$ gram of ascorbic acid there is a sharp decline of cholesterol in the blood. (2) It is possible that periodic use of ascorbic acid will prevent the development of atherosclerosis in healthy people of advanced ages. (3) Large doses of ascorbic acid under hygienic regimes produce good therapeutic results in people suffering from atherosclerosis. (4) Some patients suffering from atherosclerosis develop high blood pressure. With the use of ascorbic acid and the hygienic regime, a reduction of the blood pressure takes place and the pressure becomes normal.

Dr. Charles G. King, Director of the Nutrition Foundation and Professor of the Columbia University School of Medicine, together with his associates, discovered the same thing—namely, that vitamin C governs the rate at which cholesterol forms in the arteries. They experimented with guinea pigs. One group was given a diet that contained no vitamin C, while the second was fed with an amount of vitamin C that should be contained in a normal diet. Naturally, those that were not getting vitamin C soon developed scurvy but the amazing thing is that those guinea pigs began to show a terrific increase in cholesterol, amounting to about 600 per cent. Dr. King, in summarizing the experiment, said: "Our work shows that deficiency of vitamin C results in complex fat formation in the test animal getting out of balance."

Besides reducing cholesterol, vitamin C plays a tremendous role, directly and indirectly, in preventing or

[124]

curing heart disease generally. This vitamin maintains the blood vessels and connective tissues in good condition, preserving the strength of the capillary walls. This one function of vitamin C is of great importance in considering the underlying causes of heart disease.

Dr. Sidney G. Spector in the June, 1953 issue of the *Journal of the American Dietetic Association* says, "Almost any stress, if sufficiently severe and prolonged, will cause a lowering of the amount of ascorbic acid (vitamin C) in the tissues." He gives a few examples of what he considers *stress*. One of them is traumatic shock. Traumatic refers to a wound or injury. He then mentions "fractures and burns and in general those conditions associated with extensive tissue injury." He refers to stress as being exposed to cold, or, for example, immersing a man in cold water for eight minutes. He states that vitamin C deficiencies were noted in soldiers "subjected to the stress of arctic travel." It is interesting to note further the statement of Dr. Spector to the effect that, "In man, prophylactic or therapeutic administration of ascorbic acid heightens resistance to traumatic shock and is a valuable aid in the treatment of burns." If one has to have an operation one should prepare one's body to resist the shock of it, by taking in advance a large amount of vitamin C.

Stress, in the sense that Dr. Spector uses it, is a physical irritation of the body, but it must lead to an upsetting of the emotions, causing worries and tensions. Thus, both physical and mental stresses are closely related.

In *Metabolism,* a medical journal (1:197, 1952),

[125]

there is an account of work done by Dr. C. L. Pirani on the relationship between vitamin C and human stress. Dr. Pirani advises that, "under conditions of acute or chronic stress . . . ascorbic acid should be given in a relatively high dosage in the region of one or two grams daily during the acute stage of stress, and 300 milligrams daily thereafter." A person who has heart disease is especially vulnerable to stressful situations which may develop and should be protected by an adequate intake of vitamin C.

In the article on coronary thrombosis by J. C. Paterson, M.D., which appeared in the February, 1941 issue of the *Canadian Medical Association Journal,* the author describes a project in which 58 cases of death through coronary thrombosis were studied. It was found that in 52 of them there was a hemorrhage at the point where the clot occurred. He cites the case of another series of a greater number of cases by doctors Horn and Finkelstein in which similar results were obtained. Of the various factors that may be responsible for these hemorrhages he first discusses high blood pressure, medically known as hypertension, and he brings evidence to show that thrombosis is found more frequently in cases of chronic hypertension. Specifically he produces evidence of a study at Ottawa Civic Hospital in 1938-1940 which showed in a series of 180 cases that such hemorrhages as well as rupture of capillary walls occur five times as often in high blood pressure situations. It was also discovered that the higher the blood pressure the more frequently do hemorrhages and rupture occur.

He shows that the strength and elasticity of the capillary walls are factors in producing these hemorrhages, mentioning that incorrect nutrition may be a cause, especially a vitamin C deficiency. This is so because an insufficiency of vitamin C can result in a weakening of the capillary walls, "due to a reduction in the amount of intercellular cement substance."

He describes the extent of vitamin C deficiencies in 455 consecutive public ward patients of the Ottawa Civic Hospital in 1940, a study in which it was found that about 56 per cent of them showed a marked deficiency of vitamin C in their blood. These ward patients are persons who are of low financial status, but Dr. Paterson cites a study made by Croft and Snorf which showed that similar deficiencies existed in private patients. It was noted that significantly more deaths from coronary occlusion occurred in the winter than in the summer, although it may also be due to the fact that changes in cold periods in the winter are accompanied by increases in blood pressure.

Now, these 455 ward cases, in which 56 per cent were found to be vitamin C deficient, were cases of all kinds. But when they were narrowed down only to those who were suffering from coronary occlusion, it was found that 81 per cent were deficient in vitamin C.

Dr. Paterson states that his evidence shows that a vitamin C deficiency makes the capillary walls fragile and more easily subject to rupture, hemorrhage, and occurrence of blood clots. He says, "At the same time there is sufficient evidence to warrant the recommenda-

[127]

tion that patients with coronary artery disease be assured of an adequate vitamin C intake."

Evidence of vitamin C deficiency in the American public is given by J. B. Youmans in the *Journal of the American Dietetic Association,* (28:1029, 1952), where he says, "That too complacent an attitude in this respect (a loss of interest by the medical profession in nutritional deficiency disease) is not altogether warranted, is suggested by the recent report of Follis, Park and Jackson of a rather surprising amount of scurvy in children under two." Scurvy is caused by an insufficiency of vitamin C, and the average infant today gets plenty of orange juice.

In view of what has been shown on the subject of vitamin C, it becomes highly desirable that the entire population, down to infants, take some kind of supplementary vitamin C product, and we suggest that it be a natural product like rose hip tablets. This may be obtained in powder form and sprinkled in children's porridge, soup, etc. Rose hips contain not only vitamin C, but also the whole array of necessary minerals which are so important to the body's efficient metabolism process. Anyone suffering from no matter what form of heart disease will see at once how essential it is to add extra vitamin C to his diet.

We do not care as much for the pure ascorbic acid form of vitamin C. It is made from the sugar of maize, but contains no minerals, as do rose hip tablets.

A word of warning to heart cases: Smoking is vitamin C's greatest enemy. Every puff taken destroys some of the body's vitamin C.

An article in the *New York Times* for September 6, 1955 tells of definite research relating smoking to fatty particles in the blood.

"Men who smoke cigarettes regularly run a 40 per cent greater risk of dying of coronary heart disease than do non-smokers," says the article.

". . . the link has been established between smoking, the presence in the bloodstream of giant particles of fatty materials, and the development of coronary heart disease. This affliction is one of the leading causes of death in the nation today. Heart diseases are now the leading cause of death in the United States; coronary heart disease alone accounts for nearly half of all deaths due to heart and blood vessel diseases in general."

The September, 1955 issue of *Geriatrics* carried the article giving the original research which, incidentally, was financed by the United States Atomic Energy Commission.

A method was devised first of all for separating the fatty components from other materials in human blood serum. From these tests it was established that blood can be separated into layers of larger and smaller molecules.

It was also found that there is a relation between the abundance of larger or giant fat molecules in the blood and deaths from coronary heart disease. High fat levels mean high mortality figures.

Finally, it was found that fat levels were raised to a significant level in regular male smokers between the ages of 20 and 29. A lesser increase was found in males between 30 and 59. No correlation was found between

[129]

smoking and the presence of giant fat molecules in women. The only aspect of smoking studied was cigarette smoking—nothing was done on pipes or cigars.

The amount by which the fat molecules increased in the blood of all male subjects who smoked twenty or more cigarettes a day was enough to raise the overall death rate by 40 per cent.

Cholesterol and Choline

There are many parts of the vitamin B complex that have been shown by medical research to be of value in the prevention and cure of atherosclerosis. Choline is one of them. Choline is a lipotropic agent, which means that it combines readily with fats or oils, and thus hastens the removal of fat deposits. In the *Proceedings of the Society of Experimental Biology and Medicine* (73: 37-38, 1950) there is an article describing a study of the effect of choline on 230 patients, done by Dr. L. M. Morrison, and W. F. Gonzales of the College of Medical Evangelists, Los Angeles, Calif. It was summarized in *Modern Medicine* as follows: "Half the patients were given conventional medication but no choline after discharge from the hospital; the other half received choline daily for one to three years. Among the untreated patients, the three-year death toll was about 30 per cent, while only 12 per cent of the choline-treated patients died."

These patients were given synthetically made choline. If, however, you take brewer's yeast or desiccated liver you would be getting choline in its natural form, which is much safer. In this experiment the aim was to give

[130]

a maximum dose of 32 grams of choline daily by mouth, but many patients suffered side effects such as gastro-enteritis, dizzy spells and unpleasant body odors. They had to take doses of only 12 grams daily. By taking brewer's yeast and desiccated liver plus natural vitamin C (rose hips, etc.), there would gradually develop a condition inhospitable to an over-supply of cholesterol in the arteries, and it would be effected by natural vitamins.

Pyridoxine (Vitamin B₆)

It seems that pyridoxine is also involved in the process by which the body uses fat. In an article that appeared in *The Journal of Chronic Diseases* for July, 1955, there is an article called "Is Atherosclerosis a Condition of Pyridoxal Deficiency?" written by Henry A. Schroeder, M.D. of the Department of Internal Medicine, Washington University School of Medicine, St. Louis, Mo. In this article Dr. Schroeder tells us that too little pyridoxine in the diet of monkeys produces in general the same condition as human hardening of the arteries. He says also that a deficiency of pyridoxine in the rats causes high blood pressure. There is evidence, he says, that the whole process takes place in the blood vessels of these animals very much as it does in those of man.

Dr. Schroeder gives us an excellent estimate of the amount of pyridoxine in the average American diet. About half the pyridoxine in grain is lost when the grain is processed. Canned vegetables contain little, although fresh vegetables and fruits are quite rich in it.

[131]

The processing of milk and meat, cooking and stewing food result in substantial losses of the vitamin. Any amount of heat or light damages pyridoxine.

It is estimated that an adult may need from 2 to 3 milligrams of pyridoxine daily. Losses after processing and cooking may make it impossible for us to get enough of the vitamin, especially during winter.

"Therefore from the incomplete data in the literature, it is entirely possible that the American adult is maintained on a marginal intake of this important co-enzyme (pyridoxine) during periods of the year in which fresh vegetables and fruits are not available and processed foods and meats are widely used." Of course, too, one must take into account the quite considerable group of people who simply do not eat fresh fruits and vegetables even when they are available. Such folks would be bound to be lacking in pyridoxine the year round.

Now for the part pyridoxine plays in fat metabolism. Part of its job is to assist the body in using the unsaturated fatty acids—those important kinds of fat which occur in unhydrogenated vegetable oils and not in animal fats to any great extent. If there were a shortage of these unsaturated fats in the diet, one might need even more of the B vitamin pyridoxine than otherwise; if there were plenty of these fats in the diet, then one might need less pyridoxine. The American diet is notoriously lacking in liquid vegetable and cereal oils, especially as compared to other countries where little animal fat is eaten and liquid oils are used exclusively for cooking and for baking. We know that cholesterol, the fatty substance that collects on artery walls in hardening of the arteries, is dissolved by the unsaturated fatty acids. Dr. Schroeder also tells us that the cholesterol levels in the blood of monkeys deficient in pyridoxine is higher than that of monkeys which are getting plenty of the vitamin, which seems to indicate that pyridoxine plays a part, too, in the whole complicated business of how the body uses fats—for good or for harm.

Pyridoxine as well as choline can be assured through adequate supplies of brewer's yeast, desiccated liver and blackstrap molasses. It also comes in raw fruits and vegetables, in heart, wheat germ and peanuts.

Inositol

According to many independent medical observers, inositol, another fragment of the vitamin B complex, is concerned in some way with the metabolism of fat, as well as cholesterol. There have been numerous researches on animals as well as on people that have proven that the daily taking of the vitamin inositol will result in a lowering of the cholesterol content of the blood.

An article in *Newsweek* for September 11, 1950, describes the experiments of Dr. Louis B. Dotti, Dr. William C. Felch and Miss Stephanie J. Ilka of St. Luke's Hospital, New York, who experimented with feeding two groups of rabbits a capsule of cholesterol daily. One group of rabbits received just cholesterol and a regulation diet. The other group of rabbits got, in addition to

[133]

the cholesterol, a capsule of inositol. At the end of the feeding period the first group of rabbits showed an increase of 337 per cent in the cholesterol content of their blood. Those who had received inositol, too, showed an increase of only 181 per cent.

This same group of researchers (Felch and Dotti) in the *Proceedings of the Society of Experimental Biology and Medicine* (72: 376, 1949) describes the effect of inositol on a group of 30 diabetic patients over an 8 week period which resulted in a marked decrease in the blood of cholesterol. In a booklet of the Mellon Institute called *The Biochemistry of Inositol* there is an entire chapter with many medical references describing the effect of inositol in lowering blood cholesterol levels. There can be no question that this vitamin is an effective agent in preventing cholesterol from attaining dangerous proportions in the blood.

CHAPTER XV

Vitamins for Healthy Blood Vessels

Fifteen years of study and research have not yet succeeded in producing any satisfactory proof that cholesterol, a dominant element in all fats, is actually a cause of atherosclerosis. The disease, it is known, involves the formation of plaques of solid matter on the walls of arteries. These plaques narrow the amount of space available for the passage of blood and in time can even shut off an artery entirely. Another danger is that a chunk of arterial plaque may break away from the blood vessel wall and entirely clog a narrow point in the artery, or else flow into the heart causing a heart attack. And even though it is doubtful that cholesterol is responsible for the formation of plaque, there is no doubt that it plays some important role in arterial disease, since it is always one of the major ingredients in the plaques that are formed.

Yet it is well known that there are large numbers of people who go through entire lifetimes with what is considered unusually high levels of blood cholesterol, and still never form the deadly plaques.

What can make the difference?

A study published in Budapest in 1965 by the Hungarian Academy of Sciences gives us a clue. It suggests that this particular role of protecting against harmful effects when cholesterol level is high is played by elements in the diet, specifically vitamins A and E.

Titled "Preventive Effect of Vitamins A Plus E on The Evolution of Cholesterol-Induced Atherosclerosis," the research paper was written by three doctors, Horn, Palkovits, and Scher of the Institute of Anatomy of Budapest University School of Medicine. The paper was read at an International Conference on Gerontology held in Budapest in 1965.

Fat Deposits Prevented

The authors were intrigued by reports published in 1952 by Weitzel, a German research scientist, who found first that vitamin A protected cholesterol-fed rabbits against deposition of the cholesterol in the wall of the coronary artery, and in a later study found that vitamins A and E together were far more effective in this respect than vitamin A alone. "In consideration of the fact outlined above we have found it of interest to examine whether vitamins A and E administered simultaneously with cholesterin have any effect on the devel-

[136]

opment of atherosclerosis particularly as regards the possible preventive effect of the two vitamins. The significance of the problem is enhanced by the well-known fact which has been amply confirmed by our own observations collected for more than 25 years at the Diabetes Welfare Center—namely that the incidence of atherosclerosis in diabetic subjects is particularly high."

The authors performed their experiments with rabbits. (One does not, naturally, perform life-endangering experiments on human beings.) Dividing the animals into two groups they fed the first group large amounts of cholesterol alone, while the second group were given equal amounts of cholesterol but were also given oral doses of 50 milligrams of vitamin E and 10 milligrams of vitamin A. After sixteen days of such feeding, the animals were sacrificed and examined. It was found that the vitamins had no influence whatsoever on the increase in the blood cholesterol level of both groups. In both of them the level had risen from 88 milligrams per cent to 236 milligrams per cent.

However, and here is what is significant, the vitamins kept the fat from depositing on the arterial walls. "The essential difference as compared with the former group lies in the almost complete lipid depletion of the endothelial cells as a consequence of parallel administration of vitamins A and E."

Thus the authors confirmed the results of Weitzel and established to their own satisfaction that while these vitamins have no cholesterol-reducing effect, they do have a strong effect in preventing the actual plaque

[137]

formation that is a major portion of the disease called atherosclerosis.

Study Is Small but Important

Published with a set of color photos that demonstrate graphically the difference in the effect cholesterol can have on one's arteries depending on whether or not we are well supplied with vitamins A and E, the paper makes an interesting study out of all proportion to its small size and limited scope. It is not a pretentious study. It makes no big claims of scientific brilliance or great discovery. And yet, contained within this small scope, there may be the explanation that doctors have been seeking for fifteen years, of why high cholesterol levels are not in themselves the cause of atherosclerosis, even though they seem definitely to be a precondition for the development of the disease.

The difference is very likely in the kind of diet, or the kind of vitamin supplements that a person consumed along with the animal fats he eats. Both A and E are fat soluble vitamins and when they are carried in solution in cholesterol they may very well effect important if mysterious chemical changes in that fat. We can be reasonably sure that the vitamin E would prevent rancidity and the production of hydrogen peroxide since this is one of that vitamin's well-known effects. Can such an effect play a role in the preventing of atherosclerosis? There is so little knowledge in this area that we could not begin even to speculate on the question.

[138]

As yet we have found no indication of how this phenomenon works or why. But even without explanation, the simple fact that good amounts of vitamins A and E in the diet will protect against the formation of atherosclerotic plaque is of enormous importance. Atherosclerosis is the leading cause of heart disease and heart disease is the major killer in the United States.

Can you think of a better reason for remembering to take your vitamins daily?

Part Five:

THE HEART MUST HAVE MINERALS

CHAPTER XVI

Potassium Is Essential

Potassium is an essential mineral that is easy to forget, and whose lack may be one reason the death rate from heart disease keeps climbing so steadily in the United States. The L. Peter Cogan Foundation, of New York, recently issued a report suggesting that national heart disease rates are inversely tied to the amount of potassium in a nation's traditional foods. Where potassium-rich foods are frequently consumed (Japan, Scandinavia, Italy, France, Germany, Netherlands and Switzerland) the heart disease rates are low, compared with countries whose diets are not particularly rich in potassium (United States, Australia, Canada, New Zealand, United Kingdom.) The Japanese eat plenty of potassium in seafood and seaweed (kelp), and the potassium-rich mushrooms that appear frequently in their national dishes. Italians are fond of seafood; olive

[143]

oil and grape wine (both good potassium sources) are part of every meal.

In the *New York State Journal of Medicine* (July 15, 1967) J. Yerushalmy, Ph.D., and Herman Hilleboe, M.D., presented evidence from 22 countries showing that the presumed association between the percentage of fat calories available for consumption in the national diet and mortality from arteriosclerosis and other heart ailments is not valid. "It is true that the Japanese and Italian diets contain a much smaller percentage of animal fats than the United States. On the other hand, the diets of Swedes, Danes and Norwegians contain approximately the same proportion of animal fat as that of the Americans, but the mortality rate in these countries is just a little over a third of that in America." The Cogan Foundation report suggests that the potassium rich diet of seafoods and mushrooms consumed in the Scandinavian countries may be a mitigating factor. The report reinforces its point by showing that potassium deficiency can have a heavy influence on the ordinary workings of the heart. Dr. Samuel Bellet in his book *Potassium: Cardiac Aspects, The Role of Potassium in Health and Disease* (1952) writes, "Animals fed diets low in potassium failed to grow at a normal rate. After several weeks the heart shows evidence of myocardial necrosis.

". . . A heart lesion may be produced in four days by a diet low in potassium and high in sodium chloride, together with injections of desoxycorticosteroneacetate." A famous heart researcher, Dr. Hans Seyle of the University of Montreal, performed experiments on rats, injecting them with potassium and magnesium to

[144]

protect them against sudden extreme stress. Those not treated in this way developed damage in the heart muscle and died.

Investigators are still working to find out exactly what it could be in the potassium-rich foods that has such a beneficial influence against heart disease. One important consideration is potassium's effect on the skeletal muscles which contain about six times as much potassium as sodium. It influences the contractility of the smooth, skeletal and cardiac muscle and profoundly affects the nerve tissues. It could be that potassium's greatest contribution to heart health is its maintenance of the heart's muscle power.

Major deficiencies of potassium, so serious that they are obvious upon examination, are rare. But it doesn't take a major deficiency to cause trouble. Even minor shortages of potassium can bring on vague weakness, impairment of neuromuscular function, poor reflexes and mental confusion. The muscles become soft and saggy and healthy cell growth is sluggish, when optimum potassium is missing.

While it is true that Americans don't eat as much seafood and mushrooms and drink as much wine as the people of many countries do, there would be no problem in our getting enough potassium if our diet habits were pegged more to fresh, natural foods than the processed ones we favor. There is plenty of potassium in meats, seeds, green leafy vegetables and fruits. But the popular choices are the highly processed items. Raw peaches contain 880 milligrams of potassium per 100 grams. Can them and the reading goes down to 450. Frozen peaches contain only 133 milligrams of potassium per hundred grams. Wheat germ contains 780 milligrams of potassium per hundred grams, while self-rising, enriched, fortified, all-purpose flour has 90. The popular fig bar cookies contain absolutely no potassium, but dried figs have a reading of 780 milligrams per hundred grams.

Dr. W. A. Krehl, writing in *Nutrition in Clinical Medicine* (August 22, 1966) said, "If food habits had always been sound, the event of potassium deficiency and depletion would not have developed as a major medical problem." He affirms that poor dietary habits, restricted diet selection, misuse and inappropriate choice of foods are all to blame for any potassium deficiencies that exist.

You can go after a better potassium balance in your system by following a few simple rules. Try to be sure there is a good amount of meat in your diet every day and don't overshadow it by useless carbohydrate foods. Use salads at every opportunity along with any other fresh fruit or vegetable in season. Cut your salt intake. The sodium in salt is constantly at war with potassium for the control of the cells. When sodium takes over a poisonous condition exists that leads to death of the cells and the eventual destruction of tissues. Supplements that can provide extra potassium are bone meal, brewer's yeast, sunflower seeds, desiccated liver and wheat germ.

If maintaining a good potassium supply is indeed the key to a healthy heart, it is a goal that's easy enough to accomplish. Review your daily eating habits and take the steps necessary to improve your personal odds against getting heart trouble.

CHAPTER XVII

The Heat, Your Heart
and Potassium

Intense exposure to heat of the sun can bring on heart disease. The rhythm of the heartbeat is altered, the valves of the heart are disturbed and coronary circulation and myocardial function are abnormal in experimental animals after over-heated periods of as little as two hours. A spontaneous change in blood chemistry, and in some cases, signs of heart failure or circulatory failure characterized 44 human cases of heat stroke cited in a study by John C. Ham, M.D., and Alton M. Paull, M.D. (*Rhode Island Medical Journal,* October, 1958).

The mystery of what goes on inside, what heat exposure does to the body physiology to hurt the heart has been a subject of speculation and experimentation

[147]

among heart researchers for more than a generation. The effect of a hot climate on the body's potassium supply was examined by James L. Schamadan, M.D., and W. D. Snively, Jr., M.D., in *Industrial Medicine and Surgery* (December, 1967) and it helps greatly in clarifying the heat-heart disease relationship.

The article points out that potassium is so intimately involved with normal heart action that Drs. Sidney Franklin and Daniel Simmons of Mount Sinai in Los Angeles and the UCLA Medical School have suggested that heart trouble can be predicted from a change in the normal potassium levels. All muscles, the heart muscle included, contain especially high amounts of potassium. Schamadan and Snively demonstrate that high heat causes excessive losses of potassium, since one of the major ingredients of perspiration is potassium. So the relationship between heat exposure, heart trouble and potassium loss now becomes clearer.

The body has about 2 million sweat glands to regulate the body heat. Evaporation of the sweat from the body surface cools the blood close to the skin, then the cooler blood returns to the internal body parts where it acts to reduce body temperature. Sweat is composed of sodium chloride, potassium, ammonia and urea. When exposure to high heat is continued, the sodium and chloride content of the sweat decrease, but mysteriously the outpouring of potassium goes up to as much as three times normal.

A striking correlation between potassium deficit and heat exhaustion was noted during a prolonged heat

[148]

wave which involved the Central Great Plains and Mississippi Valley areas in July, 1966. Temperatures never went under 90 degrees Fahrenheit for three weeks and hovered above 100 degrees for more than a week. Coincidental power shortages prevented adequate air conditioning. During this time more than 150 deaths were officially attributed to "heat prostration" or "heat exhaustion." An examination of hospital records showed that many of the victims had depressed serum potassium levels.

In every case, perspiration had been excessive in the days before collapse. Many who had cardiovascular disease were taking thiazide or digitalis or both. Thiazide is known to encourage potassium losses, and coupled with excessive perspiration and a lowered potassium intake due to lack of appetite in the heat, set the stage for severe potassium deficits. Observers believe that this potassium deficit could have contributed heavily to the heat-stress disease that killed these people.

Schamadan and Snively report on other workers' findings of heart failure cases and increased incidence of heart trouble in young people in high-temperature areas who had no previous history of heart disease. The researchers feel that potassium depletion may have been the reason for heart trouble here too. When Schamadan studied heat-tolerance problems in Vietnam he noticed that two pilots showed exceptional ability to maintain high levels of performance over long periods, in spite of the heat. Both of the men consumed large amounts of ketchup with almost every meal.

[149]

Plain tomato ketchup contains quite large amounts of potassium.

What About Salt Tablets?

The article in *Industrial Medicine and Surgery* warns against overloading the system with salt when doing physical work in humid heat. Loading with sodium chloride accentuates the exchange of sodium for potassium in the kidneys and may promote heavy kidney losses of potassium.

At the 48th Annual Session of the American College of Physicians in San Francisco (April 10, 1967) R. M. Vertel and J. P. Knochel pointed out the possible relationship between potassium depletion and high incidence of heat stroke among otherwise healthy soldiers in basic training and football players in pre-season conditioning. They warned strongly against the indiscriminate use of salt tablets for the reasons listed above. They said the peasants of Indonesia and Nigeria consume daily diets high in potassium but quite low in sodium, still these people resist heat injuries characterized by electrolyte disturbances, fever, etc.

Dr. P. Prioreschi, writing in the *Canadian Medical Association Journal* (April 29, 1967), stated that while it has been established that a number of substances widely found in our environment are actively toxic to the heart, one particular mineral nutrient—potassium —was able in almost every case to counteract the effects of these poisons and prevent heart attacks.

Potassium was called a treatment for exhaustion and fatigue by Dr. P. E. Formica in *Current Therapeutic*

Research (March, 1962). He administered potassium and magnesium salts of aspartic acid to 84 housewives and 16 men who had complained of headache, insomnia, back pain, marital difficulties and boredom for weeks, some for years. At the end of the trial, 87 per cent of the subjects had responded favorably. Among other results, marital difficulties decreased. Sexual responsiveness, often diminished in middle-aged people due partly to fatigue, improved in these patients. Dr. Formica concluded that "Potassium and magnesium salts of aspartic acid, although not a panacea, afford the first fully, first truly effective physiological treatment for chronic fatigue whether or not it is associated with organic disease."

As the summer season comes on, it is particularly important to be conscious of your potassium supply. Some early symptoms of potassium deficiency are weakness and impairment of neuromuscular function, absent reflexes, mental confusion, muscles that are soft and sagging and dry skin in the mature person. In adolescents, the acne condition is considered a clarion call for more potassium.

Persons who have experienced any cardiac difficulties should be especially careful of their potassium supply. Working or even playing in the hot sun for extended periods can be a threat. Those whose jobs expose them to high heat for long periods should be especially careful about their salt intake as well as the sources of potassium in the diet.

[151]

CHAPTER XVIII

Calcium and Magnesium

That the human heart is an unbelievably efficient type of pump, able to push incredible quantities of fluid and to work continuously, day and night, without ever resting, is a phenomenon that has long been recognized. Not so long known and far from universally recognized is the fact that the mineral nutrient, calcium, is indispensable to the ability of the heart to keep working. Failure to recognize this might be compared to understanding that a gasoline explosion turns the drive shaft of a car but not knowing that the gasoline will not explode unless it has a spark plug to ignite it.

Dr. Winifred Nayler of the Baker Medical Research Institute describes the process in *Heart Journal* (March, 1967) as an electrochemical process that takes place within each cell of the heart. On the outer surface of each heart tissue cell there is a thin filament known as actin. The actin reaches with a kind of magnetic attraction toward the center of the cell, shortening its length. The result of many cells shortening at one time is contraction of the muscle. And it is calcium fed to the actin by the bloodstream, that provides both the stimulus and the means by which the actin does its work. A shortage of calcium must inevitably result in a weakened heartbeat, which can be sped up by drug stimulants but cannot be strengthened, as long as the calcium is deficient. Even this simple explanation, we believe, points out the folly of treating a weak heartbeat with drugs, at least until the ability to absorb calcium and the quantity of calcium in the diet have been checked and corrected.

To continue our analogy, however, when you understand that it takes a spark plug to ignite your gasoline, that isn't the end of the story. It also takes ignition points to direct electrical energy to the right spark plug at the right time. And as Dr. Nayler tells us, while calcium is fundamentally necessary to the heartbeat, the calcium will not do what it is supposed to do unless it is controlled in its turn by a sufficient quantity of magnesium in the system.

The reason for this, Dr. Nayler tells us, is that it is necessary for the actin alternately to absorb and release calcium. If it could not do both, the heart would either contract and stay contracted or else refuse to contract at all. To create a system in which the heart can keep contracting and relaxing alternately requires that it be a very busy living chemical laboratory. And it is magnesium that seems to be the key element that actually

[153]

regulates the heartbeat. How does it do it? By providing a tiny positive electrical charge that repels calcium, pushing it to the opposite side of the individual cell and reversing the contraction that has just taken place. Throughout the body, magnesium seems to be the mineral of basic importance in this matter of controlling the manner in which electrical charges are utilized to induce the passage of materials in and out of cells.

Nor is the heart the only portion of the circulatory system that is affected and, in effect, controlled by whether we obtain enough magnesium in our diets.

Throughout our system, all muscular tissues are designed to be able both to contract and to relax, and if either function fails there is trouble. Hypertension, or high blood pressure, is caused by an excessive contraction or inability to relax of the muscles surrounding the walls of arteries. It was reported in the *Journal of the American Medical Association* (February 22, 1965) by Dr. R. H. Seller that magnesium salts induced these muscles to relax and had therefore been found effective as a treatment for high blood pressure.

Similarly, in experimenting on the cellular metabolism with possible treatments for arteriosclerosis (hardening of the arteries), Dr. T. Shimamoto reported in the *American Heart Journal* in 1959 that he was able to reduce swelling and consequent constriction of arterial walls with magnesium salts. According to Dr. Mildred Seelig (*American Journal of Clinical Nutrition,* June, 1964) there is a direct relationship between the amount of magnesium in the diet and ability to avoid high blood pressure. Dr. Seelig regards the dif-

[154]

ference in magnesium consumption as an important reason why there are far fewer heart attacks among Orientals than there are in the West.

The study of magnesium and its many roles in human metabolism is only in its infancy. Until very recent years, this was the forgotten mineral. It was known to be essential, but nobody had any idea what it really does within the system nor did anyone seem to care much.

Today it is a different matter. As the new science of biochemistry gets under way, scientists have come to realize how important is the long-known fact that our bodies are constantly generating tiny electrical impulses and discharging them. Long regarded as a curiosity of no great significance, these minute electrical charges have been learned to be an essential part of the processes of life. Every movement, external or internal, is triggered by such impulses transmitted along nerves. Without our electrical systems, there could be no life whatsoever. And so, today, we are compelled to recognize that if magnesium is the primary regulator of the electrical activity within our bodies, then magnesium is obviously of far greater importance to health and life itself than anybody had guessed even ten years ago. This being so, what chance is there that you are getting enough magnesium in your regular diet?

Practically none unless you take special magnesium supplements, among which *Prevention* recommends dolomite as the most natural and most complete. Dr. Mildred Seelig calculated that the average American falls short by 200 milligrams a day or more of the

[155]

optimal amount of magnesium one should consume for good health. Present in many foods, magnesium is unfortunately extremely sensitive to heat and easily lost during the processing of foods. People who eat raw and unprocessed foods probably get enough. How many in America do? How many in America even find it possible?

Therein, perhaps, lies the answer of the riddle of why so many Americans get heart attacks, high blood pressure, and strokes and why these diseases are on the increase in western Europe. Nor is the circulatory system the only group of organs you will be giving a health boost if you are careful to add more magnesium to your diet. Even among essential nutrients, this one seems just a bit more essential.

The relatively new approach to heart problems—preventive cardiology—also spotlights potassium and magnesium as especially valuable for preserving the health of the heart muscle. According to Eors Bajusz, M.D., Ph.D., of Bio-Research Institute in Cambridge, Massachusetts, this area is the most common place of injury in cardiac diseases. The nutrition present there might explain why one individual has the ability to resist heart disease while another develops fatal degenerative changes in the heart muscle when he is exposed to the same stresses. The article in the *Medical Tribune* (February 29, 1968) states that apparently variations in such dietary elements as glucose, lactate, pyruvate, fatty acids and amino acids do not play a major role in determining which heart will suffer and which will not. Yet, says Bajusz, "Certain electrolytes,

[156]

especially potassium and magnesium seem to be key factors in this respect."

When fed with experimental diets deficient in one or both of these minerals, laboratory animals suffered severe disturbances in cardiac function, degeneration of myocardial fibers and cardiac death. Even today, scant attention is paid to the large number of experimental studies indicating that even a transient decrease in myocardial potassium and magnesium concentrations is of considerable importance because it generally sensitizes the heart muscle to cardio-toxic influences and, conversely, a dietary excess of K (potassium) and/or Mg (magnesium) protects the heart against the induction of morphologic abnormalities . . ." The doctor was able to demonstrate that giving these two mineral salts to laboratory animals prevented the development of 18 types of potentially fatal heart problems.

The article concludes, significantly, that a large percentage of patients admitted to hospitals reveal some degree of potassium deficiency and that in general, the average potassium intake of Americans is much lower than they think it is. "Under potentially cardio-toxic influences, the nutritional requirement of cardiac muscle cells increases as far as the need of K or Mg ions is concerned, and the customary dietary intake is insufficient to satisfy this increased demand." It is suggested that the two minerals act together to protect the heart.

More on Magnesium

In our files there are several proofs that good results in coronary cases can be obtained by the use of mag-

[157]

nesium without potassium. Here is S. E. Browne, M.D., writing to *The Lancet* (London, Dec. 9, 1961), who says that for the past 9 months he has injected a magnesium sulphate solution into patients with severe angina or a history of coronary thrombosis with excellent results in 5 patients with really severe angina.

Another piece of evidence is in an article in *The Lancet* (Nov. 1, 1958) which says, "Recent work has suggested that magnesium may be related to atherosclerosis and ischemic heart-disease. It has been claimed that magnesium sulphate is of therapeutic value in myocardial infarction, while a high magnesium diet has prevented the development of atherosclerosis in rats."

In *The British Medical Journal*, (Jan. 23, 1960), an item contains the following: "Over 100 patients suffering from coronary heart disease . . . were treated with intramuscular (injected) magnesium sulphate with only one death, compared to their findings in the previous year when, of 196 cases admitted and treated with routine anticoagulants, 60 died."

In *The American Heart Journal* (Feb., 1959) cases are described of damage to the heart by certain medication. Then in the summary appears the following: "The damage to the heart and the blood vessels, caused by the bacterial polysaccharide, was considered as a common phenomenon induced by some of the high molecular substances . . . Such damage was reduced effectively by the concurrent oral administration of magnesium chloride."

Another: In *The South African Medical Journal*,

(Dec. 20, 1958) . . . "The value of parenteral (not oral) magnesium-sulphate therapy in acute and chronic heart disease has once again been affirmed. One hundred twenty-five cases of angina have been treated by 5 workers with 66 per cent remission of pain. Sixty-four cases of acute coronary thrombosis or acute coronary insufficiency have been treated. Of these only one died in an acute attack. The great importance of early parenteral magnesium sulphate therapy in these acute cases has been stressed . . . It is suggested that in cases who have recovered from an attack of coronary thrombosis, life expectancy can be improved by combined heparin and magnesium-sulphate long-term therapy."

Finally, here is an interesting item from *The South African Medical Journal* (Oct. 18, 1958):

"In a personal communication to us Dr. Parsons writes as follows:

" 'We have completed 50 cases of patients treated with magnesium sulphate and have reported our findings in a paper to the *British Medical Journal*. We feel that this form of treatment has surpassed other forms especially in cases suffering from angina.' "

[159]

CHAPTER XIX

Millions Need More Chromium

America has been called the Chromium-Plated Society, but while we use masses of this mineral externally, within our bodies many of us are lacking in even the microscopic traces necessary to health. Test after test shows a systemic deficiency of chromium to be common among Americans, though it rarely occurs in the people of other countries. The deficiency is minute, but the effects on health can be enormous.

Until 20 years ago, presence or absence of this trace element in humans was hardly likely to come up in a nutritional discussion. Doctors had no way of measuring for it; it appeared to them that the element wasn't even present in healthy people. Newer laboratory methods have improved our powers of detection, and

[160]

we know now that chromium occurs in almost all living matter. In humans it appears in concentrations of 20 parts of chromium per 1,000,000,000 parts of blood! How can such infinitesimal amounts of any substance affect the workings of an engine as complex as the human body?

In the generation since chromium was recognized as important if not essential to life, researchers have struggled to pin-point its exact function in the system. The fact that it is present at birth in higher concentrations than at any other time in life, suggests a vital role. Indeed, several biochemical mechanisms of the cell may be dependent on chromium. Doctor Walter Mertz, chief of the Department of Biological Chemistry at Walter Reed Army Institute of Research, believes that chromium stimulates the activity of enzymes involved in man's energy metabolism. In an article in *Food and Nutrition* (December, 1966) he states that chromium plays an important role in the synthesis of fatty acids and cholesterol in the liver, an early step in glucose metabolism. Chromium is also closely related to optimal glucose utilization in experimental animals, according to Mertz.

Researchers first gauged the effect of chromium on the human system by feeding experimental mice or rats low-chromium diets. The animals' growth rates were impaired. They died significantly sooner than animals receiving even minute amounts of chromium in their drinking water. Their ability to handle sugar was often so severely disturbed that blood sugar levels

[161]

rose to a point where many of the animals excreted sugar in their urine.

At the Seventh International Congress of Nutrition (Hamburg, Germany, 1966) Doctor Mertz disclosed that the impaired efficiency of glucose metabolism in experimental animals "could be prevented by adding a few per cent of brewer's yeast, or of chromium-containing fractions of this yeast, or of trace amounts of trivalent chromium to the diet. Moreover, the fully developed deficit could be cured by one oral dose of 20 micrograms or an intravenous injection of .1 microgram chromium in the form of certain complexes."

He reported that in 3 consecutive tests, rats on low chromium diets became progressively worse in terms of their glucose tolerance until, finally, their blood sugar levels had reached the outer limits and remained essentially unchanged for an hour after intravenous injections of glucose. "On the other hand, supplementation of the deficient animals with 2 parts per million chromium in the drinking water slowly improved glucose tolerance within a period of 11 days." It is well accepted, he says, that chromium, itself, is not a hypoglycemic agent (a blood sugar-lowering factor) and is active only when insulin is present. However, the more complete the chromium deficiency in rats, the more severe the glucose tolerance impairment.

Chromium and Cholesterol

In 1954, G. L. Curran (*Journal of Biological Chemistry* 210: 765) reported on chromium's effect on the metabolism of cholesterol and fatty acids by the livers of rats. When rats were fed chromium while taking a low-chromium diet, the serum cholesterol levels remained low and, in the males, did not even go up with age. However, when the same diet was made chromium-deficient, the animals demonstrated a remarkable increase in cholesterol levels. "These experiments suggest that chromium and possibly other elements, may play a role in serum cholesterol hemostasis (blood levels)."

Further implications of the effect chromium has on the metabolism of fats showed up when the aortas of rats that died a natural death were examined for cholesterol plaques: in chromium-fed animals the incidence of plaques was 2 per cent; in chromium-deficient animals, 19 per cent. "Thus, on a nonatherogenic diet, the feeding of chromium appeared to inhibit development of such plaques," concluded H. A. Schroeder and associates, writing in the *American Journal of Physiology* (15: 1962).

A test of chromium's effect on human cholesterol levels was described in the *American Journal of Clinical Nutrition* (March, 1968) by Henry A. Schroeder, M.D. He reported on a group of institutionalized patients who each received 2 milligrams of chromium in their diets for 6 months. In two patients, no effect was observed and in 3, slight declines in the mean cholesterol levels appeared. But in 5 subjects, mean serum cholesterols declined 14.2 per cent from initial values. "The declines in the subjects are comparable to those obtained by dietary restriction of saturated fats. They occurred only after 5 months of chromium supplementation. In one outpatient taking one milligram per day,

[163]

serum cholesterol fell progressively, 26 per cent during 7 weeks."

We touched earlier on the characteristic low chromium supply of Americans. Schroeder reports that the average concentrations of chromium in each of 9 organs, except lungs, from United States males were significantly lower than in comparable subjects from the Near East and Far East. Africans generally had intermediate values; ". . . a sizable proportion of the American subjects sampled had a low or negligible quantity of chromium in their tissues, compared to foreigners. The total amounts in these organs, based on standard organ weights, indicated that African tissues had 1.9 times, Near Eastern tissues 4.4 times, and Far Eastern tissues 5 times as much chromium as did American."

Even within the United States, geographical differences have a great deal to do with chromium readings in human tissues. According to *Food and Nutrition News* (December, 1966) average tissue samples assayed from New York were 9 times higher than those from Denver, Colorado, and equally wide variations appeared to exist among tissue levels in foreign countries. "These differences may reflect different chromium intakes from food and water."

Only tiny amounts of inorganic salts of chromium are absorbed from the gastrointestinal tract when chromium supplements are given orally (probably about .5 percent of the dose). Schroeder suggests that the larger percentages of naturally-occurring chromium complexes are absorbed from foods. The chromium content of the average diet is about 200 micrograms a day or less. If we absorbed only .5 per cent, we would be

[164]

getting only 1 mircogram a day. But normal adults excrete 20-40 micrograms of chromium per liter of urine, suggesting that at least 10 to 20 per cent of ingested natural chromium is absorbed through the intestinal tract.

If we remember that chromium is essential for carbohydrate metabolism, it is reasonable to presume that carbohydrate foods in the natural state come equipped with enough chromium to help with their metabolism. But evidence shows that in refining foods chromium is removed. "Apparently there is little concentration of chromium in the endosperm (of wheat)—and in refined wheat flour—and (it) is partly removed, as are most of the other elements," Schroeder writes. "Therefore losses of chromium due to refining may contribute to deficiency, just as such losses could contribute to deficiencies of manganese, iron and zinc." White flour provides about 6.6 micrograms of chromium per 100 kcal (kilo-calories); whole wheat flour has 53 micrograms per 100 kcal.

The story with refined sugars is the same. White sugar contains little chromium, whereas unrefined raw sugars contain fair amounts. "Thus, the ingestion of refined sugar is associated with mineral amounts of that micronutrient which is necessary for the metabolism of sugar, whereas the ingestion of raw sugar carries with it presumably adequate amounts of this micronutrient. If glucose metabolizes chromium from tissue stores into the circulation, and if some of the circulating chromium is excreted, a proportion of the mobilized chromium would be lost in the urine, and in the case of chromium-poor refined sugar, not replaced . . ."

[165]

If these findings are accepted, and science does accept them, it is obvious that Americans—eating so much canned, overcooked fruits, vegetables and meats along with the heavily refined sugar and flour they love —are prime candidates for chromium deficiencies. If evidence were needed, the low American chromium ratings compared with those of other nationalities should fill the bill.

Suppose we did attempt to prevent the decline of our body chromium stores by increasing our daily chromium intake; would we derive any definite beneficial effects? *Food and Nutrition News* reports that, "Obviously, we do not know enough about the mechanism through which chromium brings about its effects to make a prediction. . . . In man, some forms of impaired glucose tolerance may be caused by a marginal chromium deficiency, and they can be expected to be responsive to chromium supplementation. It does appear from preliminary experiments that a fraction of cases with poor glucose tolerance can be improved by small daily doses of chromium. . . ."

Food and Nutrition News names unsaturated fats for high concentrations of chromium (from 300 to 600 parts per billion in corn oil and its products). Most meats range at around 100 parts per billion. Fresh fruits and vegetables have 20 to 50 parts per billion and drinking water may furnish up to 10 micrograms per liter, depending on the area. From these values, it is apparent that a regular, dependable supply of chromium, as it appears in brewer's yeast, is desirable insurance for those who wish to avoid problems with carbohydrate metabolism and high cholesterol levels.

[166]

CHAPTER XX

Better Health in a Trace of Zinc

Because of a newly discovered therapeutic effect on atherosclerosis, the trace mineral zinc may one day extend "his" life expectancy to equal that of "hers."

Such is the heartening conclusion divulged at the convention of the American Medical Association (June, 1967) by Dr. Walter J. Pories, one of the pioneers in zinc research, who presented the thesis that atherosclerosis, the disease of the arteries which is dealing devastating death blows to American males, may well be an environmental disease partly due to an easily correctable deficiency.

His first clue that arterial disease was related to deficiency of zinc came during a trace metal survey of a number of patients with different diseases at the

[167]

University of Rochester Medical Center. Hair zinc levels were examined in 25 unselected male patients. Those with atherosclerosis uniformly demonstrated low zinc values.

This finding that patients with arterial disease have low zinc levels has been confirmed by other investigators. Vallee of Harvard has reported that patients with myocardial infarctions have low zinc levels (*New England Journal of Medicine,* September, 1956). At the Minsk Medical Institute of Russia, 72 patients with atherosclerosis were found to have similarly low values of zinc, it was reported by N. F. Volkov (*Fed. Proc.,* 1963). Current studies of airmen with arterial disease and early observations in an older group at the University of Missouri also confirm the fact that patients with atherosclerosis are almost universally zinc deficient.

In the current studies on airmen conducted by Dr. Pories and colleagues, twelve patients with advanced or inoperable vascular disease have been treated, some for more than two years, with oral supplements of 220 mg. zinc sulfate—three times daily. "Though the series is small," Dr. Pories said, "we are delighted with our findings. All patients have shown considerable improvement and none has had any further vascular catastrophes or progression of atherosclerosis. More important than this nice improvement in these inoperable patients with advanced atherosclerosis, is the thesis that this illness is an environmental disease partly due to an *easily correctable* deficiency."

"The explanation is simple," says Dr. Pories, who is Chairman of the Department of Surgery for the Air

Force. "A tiny amount of zinc is present in enzymes essential to the original growth of mammalian organisms and also, it seems, to the regrowth of destroyed or damaged tissues. The effectiveness of zinc therapy in the treatment of this arterial disease is probably related to healing. Pathologists have found that the degenerative changes in the blood vessels are initiated by injury or by accumulation of fatty deposits which foster breakdown ulceration of the tissues of the blood vessels."

The healing power of zinc came to light quite by accident during studies in which wounded laboratory rats eating food contaminated with compounds of zinc, healed faster than others not getting the compound. Prompted by this revelation, Dr. Pories and his colleague, William H. Strain, Ph.D., tested the effectiveness of zinc on surgical patients at Wright-Patterson Air Force Base in Ohio. They gave daily capsules of zinc sulphate to ten young airmen who were undergoing a type of surgery that is always slow to heal. The rate of healing proved three times better in patients getting zinc. No toxic effects were observed in tests ranging from 43 to 61 days.

The effective role played by zinc in the healing of arterial lesions, when considered in the light of the geography of atherosclerosis, lends considerable weight to the suggestion that mineral imbalance may well be a strong causative factor and that this disease is not necessarily the inevitable concomitant of growing old. "Although vascular disease is a frequent finding in an older person," says W. C. Manion (Aging Circulation, *Mil. Med.,* July, 1963), "it should not be assumed that

[169]

vascular disease is a natural and normal sequence of aging."

If atherosclerosis were merely a degenerative disease and not related to environment, it should be evenly distributed across the United States in proportion to the aging population. This is not the case. Indeed, centenarians have been reported where careful examination has shown little or no vascular disease, while other patients have been presented with severe sclerotic lesions in the first few months or years of life (H. Hirsch, cited by Korenshevsky, *Physiological and Pathological Ageing,* Basel, Switzerland, 1961).

The environmental factor is further borne out by the fact that in some countries atherosclerosis is a rarity while in the United States it has reached epidemic proportions, eventually killing three out of every four males. Even within the United States, there are large geographic differences in the death rates from cardiovascular disease. In the surveys of the U.S. Public Health Service, it has become apparent that the highest death rates are near the two sea coasts, the Gulf of Mexico, the Great Lakes, and along the Mississippi Basin. It appears that the high death rates are associated with areas of high water drainage, where the minerals have been leached from the soils or where compounds, washing down with the rivers, could be binding minerals into a biologically unavailable form, Dr. Pories said.

In an attempt to explain the regional variations, investigators in Japan, Great Britain and the United States have pointed out that areas with soft water

[170]

have significantly higher cardiovascular death rates than areas where the drinking water contains more mineral matter.

Minerals are also leached from the soils in the presence of artificial fertilizers and poisonous sprays, says Dr. Andre Voisin in his book *Soil, Grass and Cancer*.

In fact, the Trace Element Committee of the Council on Fertilizer Application has identified 32 of the 50 states as zinc deficient. Many of these have been shown to be the high mortality states in a United States Public Health Service Survey.

The zinc deficiency of the soil is carried over to our food plants, and to the cattle which man depends upon for the staff of life. Add to this soil and water deficiency the fact that, like every other mineral element, zinc is concentrated in the bran and germ portions of cereal grains—the parts that are removed in the refining process—and not replaced in the so-called enriching program—and you have some understanding of why atherosclerosis is becoming a national tragedy.

High Zinc Foods

Food	Parts Per Million of Zinc
Barley	27
Beef	20-50
Beets	28
Cabbage	2-15
Carrots	5-36
Clams	20

[171]

Corn	25
Eggs, dry, whole	55
Egg yolk	26-40
Herring	700-1200
Liver, beef	30-85
Milk, cow	4-30
Oatmeal	140
Oysters	1600
Pumpkin seeds	38
Peanut butter	20
Peas	30-50
Rice	15
Spinach	3-9
Sunflower Seeds	66
Syrup, maple	52-105
Wheat bran	140
Yeast, brewer's	80

CHAPTER XXI

Vanadium Protects the Heart

Scientists aren't sure whether vanadium keeps excessive cholesterol from forming, or breaks it down when it has formed; perhaps it does both. The question came to the fore when researchers discovered vanadium abundant in the hard drinking waters of certain areas of the southwest, the very areas where death rates from degenerative heart disease are lowest in the United States. It is barely present in the soft water of the Coastal and Great Lakes States, the states, as the researchers suspected, where death rates from heart disease are highest. In a speech to the American Association for the Advancement of Science (December 29, 1961) Dr. William H. Strain suggested that "There are very significant geographical variations in death rates for all causes and for cardiovascular diseases that may be due to variable intake of trace elements, especially vanadium and zinc."

[173]

A great deal has been written about the possibility that all life originated in the oceans, billions of years ago. If this is true, the role of sea minerals in the physiology of man deserves more attention. In his book, *Sea Within* (Lippincott), W. D. Snively makes the point that the extra-cellular fluid (about 30 per cent of the human body) is essentially diluted sea water. Of course the body has its own mechanisms for keeping the composition of this inner ocean constant, but deficiencies of various sorts can develop when there are dietary shortages of specific minerals.

A 1956 study of the Scandinavian countries showed that the death rate from heart disease among these countries is exceptionally low. Scientists researched all types of data about these rich diet nations, trying to find an explanation for this happy state. Consideration of the consumption of fat, meat and milk in each country showed no relationship of these food factors to the death rate. The doctors found that one environmental influence that might vary is the intake of trace elements.

In sea-side Scandinavian countries, ocean fish are eaten in large quantities and sea salt (rich in a variety of trace elements) is used for preserving fish, for cattle and for household consumption. To add credibility to the importance of the water-surrounded situation of these countries, Professor Niels Dungal reported in 1953 on 2,200 autopsies in Iceland. The arteries of the Icelanders, at age 60, compared well with the arteries of Austrians at age 40. Strain suggests that their lack of cholesterol accumulation might be credited to the ingestion of vanadium and other trace minerals.

[174]

Lack of trace elements in the soil is common to certain parts of this country. The drinking water varies from very hard to very soft, and then the mineral constituents of hard water vary from place to place as well. Milk, frequently mentioned as a source of trace minerals, reflects both the soil and water that make up the environment of the cow, and its mineral composition is extremely variable. Vanadium is not present in meat in measurable amounts, but it is found in varying quantities in vegetables.

Marine life is the most reliable source of vanadium, in Dr. Strain's opinion. Particularly good sources are herring and sardines. Larger fish show variations in the content of vanadium. However, it seems reasonable that "All ocean fish contain some vanadium, but . . . the amount varies with the species."

Circulatory disturbances are frequently caused by a pile-up of cholesterol in the blood vessels. But cholesterol is a valuable constituent of the brain, spinal cord and other portions of the nervous system; so the need is to regulate cholesterol formation rather than to inhibit it completely. Presumably when the body has the proper equipment, it manages this regulation very nicely. Vanadium is part of this natural regulating system. Researchers have demonstrated that the presence of vanadium in the brain inhibits cholesterol formation. They have also shown that the formation of cholesterol in the human central nervous system can be cut by administering vanadium orally.

J. T. Mountain and associates reporting in *Federation Proceedings* (18, 425, 1959) described an elabo-

[175]

rate study with rabbits that showed vanadium added to the standard diet at premeasured levels lowered free cholesterol and fat content of the liver in the rabbits. When vanadium was added to a 1 per cent cholesterol diet, it held down the elevation of free and total cholesterols in the plasma; when rabbits were fed cholesterol to raise the plasma level, and then the cholesterol was omitted from the diet, the presence of vanadium in the diet was given credit for a faster return to normal cholesterol readings than occurred when no vanadium was furnished. Mountain and his associates concluded that vanadium both inhibits the formation of cholesterol and speeds the destruction of it.

The use of vanadium in humans for limiting the cholesterol count has been considered both as a preventive and as a type of therapy. G. L. Curran and R. L. Costello reported in the *Journal of Experimental Medicine* (103, 49, 1956) that six weeks of administering vanadium resulted in statistically significant lowering of the serum total and free cholesterol levels. The vanadium lowered tissue cholesterol stores in 4 out of 5 men studied. A small group of vanadium workers were observed, and, compared with a control group, the workers had a significantly lower cholesterol value.

It is interesting that scientists found it difficult to decide on a simple, reliable method for measuring vanadium levels in man. Although 90 per cent of ingested vanadium is eliminated in the urine, determining the urinary levels of vanadium in large communities is impracticable. A simpler method recently presented itself. Changes in the levels of vanadium show up in

[176]

the hair. Strain is hopeful now, with this simple means of measurement, that a more elaborate program for studying the important relationship between vanadium intake and cardiovascular death will be undertaken.

Dr. Strain points out that an overdose of vanadium, even in a synthetic form, is difficult to get. But *Prevention* believes that all nutritional elements, including vanadium, should be taken in the form that nature provides. Fish, of course, is an excellent source. Unfortunately, few Americans make fish any part of the diet and if they do it is too occasional to be dependable. As we have seen, milk and vegetables are also unreliable sources of vanadium, because the content of this mineral varies from one location to the next, one cow or plant to the next. It is revealing to see, then, that seaweed is frequently on the menu in the Scandinavian countries, the same ones that have such a good record for controlling heart disease. Seaweed, preferably kelp, is an ideal source of vanadium and other important trace minerals.

The brown seaweeds are the commonest, and the ones used most widely for food. Just like other plants, they contain carbohydrates, protein and other nutrients. There is some vitamin A and some of the B vitamins, but the vitamin C content of seaweed is comparable to that of many vegetables and fruits. For many Eskimos, seaweed was once the chief source of vitamin C. One test showed a vitamin C content of 5 to 140 milligrams per 100 grams of wet seaweed. Oranges contain about 50 milligrams per 100 grams.

But the main attraction of seaweed is its mineral con-

[177]

tent. Plants that grow on land take up minerals from the soil. The same is true of sea plants, and the sea is the richest source of all minerals. W. A. P. Black, writing in the *Proceedings of the Nutrition Society of England* (Vol. 12, page 32, 1953) tells us that the ash of seaweed may be from 10 to as high as 50 per cent. This means that if you burn seaweed you may have half the volume of the seaweed left as minerals. Compare this to some other foods: carrots leave an ash of 1 per cent; apples have a mineral ash of .3 per cent; almonds, 3.0 per cent. Black writes, "It can be said that seaweed contains all the elements that have so far been shown to play an important part in the physiological processes of man. In a balanced diet, therefore, they would appear to be an excellent mineral supplement."

Don't leave your mineral nutrition to chance. Scientists have proven that you need vanadium. Make sure you get it by eating all the fish you can, or, to play safe, put some kelp in your daily diet.

Part Six:

THE ROLE OF
EXERCISE

CHAPTER XXII

You Must Exercise

J. I. Rodale

The subject of exercise is so important to a heart case and to people who would like to prevent heart disease that I will go into the subject quite extensively. I have not only learned from my own experience how one can save one's life through daily exercise, but have found a terrific amount of information in the medical literature regarding the value of taking daily exercise.

There was a time when I used to pooh-pooh its value, and used to tell the story of Chauncey Depew, the famous financier of the last century, who lived to be way over 90, and who always deprecated the importance of taking exercise. "The only exercise I get," he used to say, "is to act as pallbearer for friends who used to take exercise."

[181]

Perhaps he didn't take exercise as such, but I'll wager he was a big walker, for those were the days before the auto was known. He was a stockholder in many corporations and was known to attend many board meetings, going from one to another, sometimes merely to show his face and to collect the director's fee. But there is a reason why some persons live to 90 without exercise, and why others die at 50. It is a matter of the vitality endowment at birth, the condition of the glands, chest expansion, width of arteries, etc. If a man has chosen the right ancestors, and received a good share of their physical perfection through the accident of birth, then he can break many health rules and still live to a ripe old age.

Mark Twain was another exercise scoffer. He used to say, "Whenever I feel like exercising, I lie down until the feeling passes." But Mark Twain became very sick and died before his time. He no doubt did not have the physical endowment of Chauncey Depew.

One need not spend hours in daily calisthenics. Walking furnishes a very interesting form of exercise, although at least 10 minutes of daily setting-up exercises can be very valuable. I strongly recommend a walk of at least an hour a day. Some people seem to forget that they have feet. They forget that there is such a thing as walking. The other day in visiting a hospital I walked down two flights of stairs, and a nurse remarked, in amazement, "Are you *walking* down?"

A doctor in a medical journal says, "The popular picture of the coronary heart disease victim is that of a burly business or professional man, fat and soft from over-eating and lack of exercise." Another expresses it this way, "Motion is the essence of life. Like all things pertaining to life, we know little concerning it. It is an inherent characteristic of all animate things to move through space with ease and power, not only for protection but for the pleasure of doing so." I have learned to love my daily hour's walk, and wouldn't miss it for anything except rain or snow. In fact, I'm arranging, beginning this year, to spend my winters in Florida so that I can walk all year round.

Dr. Paul D. White, the President's heart specialist, told a House Appropriations Subcommittee, "Coronary thrombosis is an epidemic. . . . Wise exercise is one remedy."

As Elbert Hubbard said, "The mintage of wisdom is to know that rest is rust, and that real life is in love, laughter and work." But today the sleeping pill is the symbol of our sedentary age. People can't sleep because they do not tire themselves out by enough movement during the day. They spend hours slumped in front of their television sets. The man who created the internal combustion chamber that furnished the activating power for the automobile killed millions of people before their time. How can we undo the auto? The instinct of the bear in his cage tells him that he must walk up and back. But man in his cage has a blunted instinct. Even doctors who should know better violate this important rule. That is why doctors have 12 times as high a death rate from angina pectoris as farm workers.

As far as I'm concerned, I'm conscious of the fact

[183]

that I have to move about as much as possible, in order
to keep the fat out of my heart muscle. I have my
telephone at another desk. Every time it rings I have
to walk 15 feet to it and 15 feet back. My office is on
the 3rd floor and every day I walk up and down to
and from it at least 4 or 5 times—sometimes more,
because I purposely do not have a buzzer system. When
I want to talk to one of my people I go to them. I do
not make them come to me.

There is too much sitting in this civilized world of
ours. Cotton Mather in his book *Angel of Bethesda,*
1724, said, "Scriveners, Tailors, and others sit still, with
little Motion of their Bodies, in the Work of their
Hands, must think of frequent Exercise, to stir their
Limbs. Be sure, Students and Men that lead sedentary
lives, will do well to be on Horseback, as much as
they can."

John Homans, M.D., in *The New England Journal
of Medicine,* January 28, 1954, said, "The prolonged
sitting position occasions a degree of dependency stasis
that may result in the rapid development of a quiet
type of thrombosis in the deep veins of the calf. From
this, a propagation of clot and pulmonary embolism
may immediately follow. . . . Such matters are important enough to suggest the advisability of making
movements of the toes, feet and lower legs when one
is sitting for long periods and of getting up and exercising when opportunity offers. The right leg seems
more susceptible than the left. There is evidence that
persons over fifty years of age should have this particularly in mind and that physicians should be alert to

[184]

recognize the significance of lameness after airplane flights, automobile trips and other occasions of a prolonged seated position."

At the theater always take a walk during intermission.

I would like to present a letter that Dr. Bernard E. Myers of London sent to the *British Medical Journal* and which was published in its July 31, 1954 issue:

"Sir,—Recently I went on a cruise to the Mediterranean and was appalled that two people died from heart complaints, one of whom was buried at sea. Another heart case had to be put ashore at Naples for hospital treatment. In addition, at least five other patients spent most of the cruise in the ship's hospital, of whom four were heart cases and one had a lung condition. Obviously, patients so severely ill are a great worry and anxiety to the ship's doctor, and depressing to other passengers. The doctor informed me that investigation has shown in many such instances that heart cases have been advised by their doctors to go on a cruise for the benefit of their health, but what of the danger and the sorrowing relatives on board?—I am, etc."

This doctor overlooks the fact that there is so much sitting about on these cruises.

If you have to do a lot of sitting at home, a good way to do it is in a rocking chair. Rocking counteracts all the disadvantages of ordinary sitting and is a pleasant activity. It also stirs up the liquid in the spine and is an aid in the prevention of the petrification of the back. But don't look at television in a rocker, unless

[185]

you can make the television set move in the same rhythm as the rocker. I tried it and after several months began to experience trouble with my eyes.

Dr. Laurence E. Morehouse, professor of physical education at the University of California, said that the human body was built for the rigors of the hunt, and when the body's connective tissue is not exercised, it shortens and thickens, causing pressure on nerves, producing sensitivity and pain and upsetting the endocrine balance. "Movements of skeletal muscles in man," he says, "not only performed his external work in primitive days, but also acted as supplemental heart muscles in moving fluids through the body.

"The modern sitting man relies on his heart muscles alone to pump the fluids which support the internal environment of the body. The heart cannot do the job of circulation without the aid of other muscle pumps and sitting man soon begins to suffer."

Dr. Edward P. Luongo of Los Angeles in a report to an American Medical Association convention described a study of 100 heart cases in the 40-to-50-year-old age group, and stated that 70 of them showed no regular exercise patterns either at work or away from their jobs. Dr. Charles H. Bradford, at an Eastern regional meeting of the International College of Surgeons in 1957, said that "Nature did not intend the intricate cardiac mechanism to serve a sedentary body. Certainly, the stimulus of natural exercise plays a wholesome part in regulating metabolic disorders."

Dr. E. R. Tretheave, of the Department of Physiology, University of Melbourne, writing in the May

[186]

12, 1956 issue of *The Medical Journal of Australia* says, "The cardiac patient, if he does not exercise himself within the limits of his heart's performance, finds his cardiac muscle is not favored thereby. It is also becoming recognized by some medical observers that the sedentary life in itself may be a contributory factor to certain cardiac illnesses."

Dr. N. E. Chadwick, health officer of the city of Hove, England, claims that the increasing speed and strain of modern life is wrongly blamed for illnesses and early death. Insecurity, in some form, he says, has been present with every generation, but today's killer is inactivity.

Dr. Burgess L. Gordon of Philadelphia dogtrots each morning to his train and walks briskly to his appointments. "It's the habit of taking things easy most of the time and then placing a sudden strain on the body in an emergency that is dangerous."

Dr. Roy M. Keller, *Journal of Medical Physical Research* (Sept., 1953) says, "Inactivity does not utilize energy, and causes a damming back to the liver and a lowering of differentials (electric) and impaired function. Utilization of energy in the body is one situation in which one can eat his cake and keep it too." We must use or lose.

Dr. W. Pinnington Jenson in *The Lancet* of June 19, 1954: Cardiovascular wear and tear is associated with the 7 fat years rather than the 7 lean ones, and the 7 fat years do not mean merely increased fat percentage of total calories, but increased percentage of

[187]

mechanical transport, sedentary occupation, and nervous as opposed to physical exertion."

Dr. Joseph W. Still of George Washington University School of Medicine: "In our advice to the aged I believe we should generally emphasize activity, rather than rest. My observation is that older people tend to be too sedentary and I think this tendency must be combatted."

Many physicians advise their patients against climbing stairs. Except in rare cases, according to the best opinion today, this is a great blunder. In a recent issue of Bernarr MacFadden's *Joyous Life* (Dec., 1954) MacFadden says, "When President Harding was serving as a Senator, he signed a testimonial which we published in *Physical Culture Magazine,* in which he stated that he cured his heart trouble by climbing stairs."

I am a heart case and as I have said a few moments ago, I climb two flights of stairs 4 or 5 times every day, and have hardened myself because of it. I can now accomplish it without becoming winded. So many of my visitors come up to my office puffing terribly. It is a sign that they don't exercise every day.

Some years ago I visited a man who wanted to show me some paintings that were on the second floor of his home. He crept up the stairs on his hands and knees. I was informed that he was a heart case. I met him recently and commented about it, and he replied that he no longer did it. Evidently some one had put a scare into him.

Frederick Othman in his column in *The N. Y. World*

Telegram (July 17, 1956) mentions a bill in the Senate to appropriate almost two billion dollars, part of which, or $50,000, was for the purpose of building an elevator in the federal courthouse at Anderson, South Carolina, which is a two-story building. Senator Paul H. Douglas, Democrat of Illinois, demanded, "Am I to understand that the judges in South Carolina are so infirm that they can't climb a flight and a half of stairs?"

Quoting Mr. Othman: "The gentleman from South Carolina said he meant that the judges' doctors had recommended that they go easy on stair-climbing. This is hard on the judicial heart beat. 'Some new judges might be cheaper than a $50,000 elevator,' snapped Sen. Douglas."

As you see, some doctors are still suggesting no stair-climbing. And in New York they are clamoring for electrical escalators for all subway stations, which is part of a growing movement for reducing our daily quota of exercise and which is going to shorten our lives. Dr. Richard T. Smith, director of the Department of Rheumatology, of the Pennsylvania Hospital, recently said that human life may well be shortened below its potential by lack of both physical and mental activity. He said, "The heart is a muscle and must have maintenance of tone. It is not the athletic heart that kills us, but lack of it."

The fact that life can be prolonged by exercise is described by Dr. Raymond Pearl, the famous Johns Hopkins researcher, in his book, "The Biology of Death," (page 212). An experiment was performed

[189]

with rats. The group that exercised lived longer than one that led a sedentary existence.

In spite of all this evidence that our national inactivity is very harmful, little is being done to remedy it. But articles are beginning to appear with titles such as "Lack of Physical Fitness in U. S. Blasted by Government Official," "Muscular State of the Union," "Nation of Softies," "Nutrition Expert Bemoans Our Horror of Exercise," "N.Y.U. Head Decries Lack of Exercise," etc., etc., etc.

Fears Loss of Essential Vitality

Shane McCarthy, executive director of former President Eisenhower's Council on Youth Fitness, said recently, "The tremendous aptitude for inactivity among Americans might end in a human erosion that could strip the nation of its strength within the next generation." Speaking at the Eastern College Athletic Conference, on December 13, 1956, he said that over 34 per cent of the draftees examined in October were rejected because they lacked physical fitness. Talking about his own sons, he said, "They all share one ambition. That is to become 16 so they can sit behind the wheel of an automobile."

In a test of the physical condition of American children as against those in Italy and Austria, 78 per cent of the Americans failed whereas only 8½ per cent of the Europeans could not pass. College freshmen have been becoming taller, but more lacking in endurance. This tendency in our youth to move less is bound to result in more heart disease when they grow up.

[190]

Is this enough? I can give you much more on the dangers of a sedentary life, but there are more aspects of the general subject of exercise which will have to be covered. So, whether you have heart disease or not, get out and move. Walk, do setting-up exercise, go window-shopping—any kind of movement will suffice. You will never regret it.

CHAPTER XXIII

More Value in Rhythmic Exercise

It is by now well-known and generally accepted that the health of the heart can be greatly affected by what we eat and how much of it. Any doctor will tell you that the avoidance of overeating and maintaining a normal weight is important to heart health. Some physicians maintain that cholesterol in the diet should be reduced while others, with whom we agree more completely, advise the reduction or elimination of sugar. While this is an important scientific controversy, as a practical matter it is merely an academic question since sugar and cholesterol usually go hand-in-hand in our foods; and reducing the intake of one is almost a guarantee that the intake of the other will also be reduced. So the medical profession really knows a great deal about how to control the diet for the sake of healthier hearts.

What is new and still controversial is the role of exercise in the regimen to promote healthy hearts. In this respect, a notable step forward was taken in October of 1966 when the Canadian Medical Association sponsored a massive symposium on "Physical Activity and Cardiovascular Health," held in Toronto and attended by hundreds of top cardiologists from all over the world. This symposium made it apparent that what had once been considered an isolated medical fad is now backed by an enormous body of research and established fact, and that what was considered dubious and questionable only a few years ago is rapidly becoming irrefutable. At any age and in any condition of health, even after a heart attack, exercise is good for the heart and the more sensible exercise a person takes, the more the heart will benefit by it.

Heart Muscle Benefits

Contrary to earlier medical belief that it is dangerous to tax the damaged or aging heart, the hundreds of experts gathered in Toronto produced extensive studies to demonstrate that the heart, like all other muscles, becomes stronger as we use it harder and place greater demands upon it. They also found that without exercise, the muscle tissue of the heart actually degenerates and shrinks away, thus making the individual more vulnerable to heart disease as well as reducing the ability of the heart to help the body withstand other diseases.

[193]

This, however, is what we have been hearing from Dr. Paul Dudley White, Dr. Joseph Wolffe, Dr. Wilhelm Raab and others for many years. What we consider the most important new development was a lengthy and enlightening study from the University of Edinburgh in Scotland, reported by A. R. Lind and G. W. McNicol. This is the first study we are aware of that has actually unveiled some of the mechanism within us by which exercise leads to changes in the muscle structure and in the circulatory system. On the basis of this study, it should be possible to make a more accurate determination than ever before of just which exercises will be of greatest benefit to the heart, and why.

Sustained Contractions

Lind and McNicol, on the basis of the knowledge they have gained, have divided exercise into two chief types: sustained contractions and rhythmic or dynamic exercise. Sustained contractions are those that involve a continuously exerted tension. Running would be a good example. When you run, you run continuously without pause for rest. Bicycle riding is similar in nature. These exercises have been recommended by some very important cardiologists on the general theory that such exertions require a great blood supply to the muscles being used, compel the heart to work harder, and result in a strengthened heart and increased lung capacity as well.

The theory would seem generally correct, yet Lind and McNicol find one serious flaw in this type of exercise. They say that: "During a contraction, the muscle's blood vessels dilate but that the increased flow of blood through the dilated vessels is opposed by the mechanical compression of the contracting muscle fibers." In other words, the blood vessels of the muscle expand to permit an increased flow of blood, but the muscle itself also swells up, compressing the blood vessels and making it harder for the blood to get through to the muscle fibers. They go on to say that "During sustained contractions the mechanical compression is unremitting and thereby presents a continuous impediment to the blood flow of the muscle . . ."

As a result, they have found, this type of exercise that they have labeled "sustained contractions" can supply the muscles being used with increased blood only by a great increase in the rate at which the heart beats and a similar rise in the blood pressure. A further result is long-lasting fatigue, with the muscle taking several hours to recover its full functional ability.

Rhythmic Exercise

The above is not to say that there is any reason why a healthy person should not take such exercise. But it is obvious that if the heart is already damaged or the general health is bad, a sudden sharp rise in blood pressure and prolonged fatigue will not be the best medicine. In contrast to such exercise, Lind and Mc-Nicol offer what they have learned about the body's way of responding to what they call "rhythmic or dynamic exercise." This is exercise in which there is an alternation between effort requiring a contraction of a set of muscles and relaxation. They point out that while the muscle contractions still restrict the blood flow to the muscles, there is a "compensatory high blood flow during the periods of relaxation. The heart rate and cardiac output can increase greatly but the blood pressure shows little or no change; the fall of peripheral vascular resistance allows the perfusion of the active muscles with no need to evoke a rise of blood pressure."

What Lind and McNicol would call a rhythmic exercise is one like rowing, in which you rest after each stroke of the oars, or a game like tennis where there is a period of relaxation after each effort. Football would be considered a rhythmic exercise, in contrast to basketball in which the action is continuous.

We consider this separation of exercise into two distinct categories an important one. Either type will cause the heart to work harder, increase its size and strength, and increase the volume of blood that it is able to handle. But for those in delicate health, it seems obvious that the rise in blood pressure that goes along with sustained contractions may be a possible hazard that it might be well to avoid. For anybody, to take hours longer to fully recover from the fatigue of exercise is an undesirable consequence.

CHAPTER XXIV

Walking Is Good for Everyone

J. I. Rodale

The historian George Macaulay Trevelyan once said, "I have two doctors, my left leg and my right"—a very witty statement, but powerfully true. In the case of a heart condition, these two doctors can save the life of the patient. Movement, that's what a heart case needs. Keep the heart pumping and teach it to like it.

People have said to me, "I'm so busy, when will I have the time to walk?" Squeeze the time out somehow. Everything else will get done, you will see. Here is an interesting plan for the beginning walker. Start off by walking 15 minutes before going to work. Then do 15 minutes during the lunch period, and 15 minutes before or after the evening meal. Slowly these periods can be lengthened until one finds that he is doing 2 hours a day without any trouble at all.

If there is something about your kind of heart condition that you think contraindicates walking, you will know it after your first 15 minutes. But it would be best to clear it with your doctor first—and then follow some kind of plan.

At the beginning it would be best to search out a flat terrain, otherwise heart cases will experience angina symptoms. Expect also that you will have more difficulty at the beginning of a walk than in the second half. If pressure pains occur, rest a moment or two. At the beginning of muscular exertion, time is required for the adjustment of the circulation to the increased oxygen demand. But this initial period of oxygen deficiency soon passes. The taking of vitamin E, which increases the oxygenation of the body, is very helpful to walkers.

There's a great advantage to heart cases in walking regularly, rather than merely at weekends. Give the heart a daily treatment. It is just like taking vitamins —you must do it every day. The cumulative effect on the heart's action will soon be noticeable. After a while you will develop a kinesthetic sense, that is, a sense of sure-footedness, a sense of perception of muscular movement. It will create grace in the motions of the body.

A great advantage in walking is perspiring. When I talk "walk" to some women, they reply that they walk plenty in the kitchen, but the trouble is they rest and sit too much in between movements. There isn't the

[198]

amount of perspiring that occurs towards the end of a steady one hour's walk. The same thing applies to men who work in factories or department stores. If you don't perspire, you aren't getting enough movement. By the sweat of thy brow shalt thou keep the heart functioning efficiently.

In an old issue of *Good Health* (Battle Creek, Mich.) I find the following: "Among civilized people the skin is almost universally anemic; that is, it does not contain the normal amount of blood, its vessels being contracted and sometimes shriveled and withered as the result of lack of use.

"Vigorous sweating has the effect to fill the skin with blood, which is capable of holding one half or two thirds of the total amount contained in the body. This filling of the skin vessels naturally withdraws a great quantity of blood from the vessels of the internal organs, and so relieves the chronic congestion which often exists in the inner parts because of inactivity of the skin, the result of wearing clothing and avoiding contact with the sun and air, which man's primitive ancestors enjoyed . . . For the maintenance of normal health, the skin should be brought into free exercise with profuse sweating at least once every day."

The body can get rid of a lot of poisonous wastes through the perspiration of the skin. It can increase its oxygen consumption, for man receives some of his oxygen through the skin, but when the skin is moist through perspiration, the amount of oxygen taken in increases. The sweating process was developed in the body for highly important purposes, and it is advisable

[199]

that that function be exercised every day. So much for perspiration.

A recent experiment performed with human subjects at the University of Aberdeen (Scotland) is of great interest in connection with walking. It deals with the effect of walking on the coagulability of the blood. A thrombosis, or a blood clot, that completely blocks the circulation in an artery, can cause death. This can come about easily. The coagulability of the blood, or the ease with which it clots, differs in different people, based on various factors. In many researches it has been shown that blood coagulability, measured by its clotting time, increases in approximately equal degree after eating a meal that is heavy with fat. In the experiment to which I refer (*The Lancet,* Sept. 20, 1958) the effect of physical activity on the increase in blood coagulability following the ingestion of a high-fat meal was studied.

Twenty-three medical students were observed over a period of days. They were given a breakfast each day very high in fats (2½ oz. bacon, 2 eggs, 1-1½ oz. butter, bread, and tea with milk and sugar). On certain days they were sedentary in their activities, while on others they walked for 3 miles. On the days when they walked it was found that the blood clotting time increased significantly, which means that it would take longer for a blood clot to form which is a very desirable thing.

This fact, namely, the lengthening of blood-clotting time by exercise, and the creation of additional veins and capillaries by exercise, are terrific arguments for doing a lot of walking each day. It will pay off in many years of extra life.

For many heart cases it is difficult to walk with comfort in the winter time. The cold constricts the arteries. There is more angina and general discomfort on cold days, and snowy time is even worse because of the combined effect of the dampness with the cold. In such cases I have resorted to my electrical indoor bicycle, and have even walked on the track of indoor gymnasiums. When walking gets into your blood, you crave it like a drug.

I have noticed an interesting thing about my walking in the cold. Instead of taking off weight, it tended to increase it. When I saw my weight actually being a little higher at the end of an hour's walk in the cold than it was at the beginning, I discontinued walking outside on very cold days. I wondered whether the body has some mechanism which protects it against the cold, perhaps by forming more fat.

I was surprised, therefore, when later I read something in a medical journal that confirmed my thinking. In the *Journal of the American Medical Association* (Dec. 30, 1950, page 1590) appears the statement, "It is concluded that cold stimulates fat metabolism."

According to the *Practitioner,* Dec. 1953, "All forms of coronary pain will occur more often in January than in July . . . It is during the winter months that hospital wards are overburdened with such cases." This affects people with poor circulation, for one reason or another.

The Lancet, Aug. 3, 1957, advises that "The blood pressure of some healthy people rose when they were

[201]

suddenly exposed to cold. The rise was accompanied by a . . . little change in pulse rate. Taken together, these changes probably increase the work of the heart. They may together explain why exposure to a cold wind excites anginal pain, and they are a possible reason why people have died suddenly on immersion in cold water."

According to a statistical study made by the Metropolitan Life Insurance Company, coronary attacks reach a high point in February of each year. Dr. George M. Wheatley of the Metropolitan recently said, "Some people feel fine in climates where there is snow and bright sunshine." There are many people, says Dr. Wheatley, who can stand sharp changes in temperature, but there are others, especially those whose small blood vessels (capillaries) do not expand and contract readily, who are in danger. Elderly people especially come into this category. I believe that this condition also affects people who have narrow arteries.

Women can stand cold better than men because they have a thicker layer of fat under the skin. Their heat loss is about 10 per cent less than that of men under the same conditions.

There is evidence that a sufficiency in the body of vitamins A, B, C, D and E is effective in enabling the body to withstand the ravages of cold.

How about walking in city streets which are polluted with gasoline and chimney vapors? If the country or large parks are not available, I walk in the city, but would take large doses of rose hip vitamin C and desiccated liver. These are known to aid the body in

[202]

getting rid of toxic substances. If you have a highly nutritious diet, if you avoid the dangerous things like sugar, factory chemicalized foods, etc., if you indulge in plenty of walking and do everything possible to harden your body and make it healthy, the polluted air will not hurt you . . . much.

When I walk in Allentown, I have worked out routes that take me for the most part through narrow alleys, where there is very little auto traffic or gasoline odors.

In walking keep your head up, don't drag your feet on the ground, and do not keep your feet too far apart.

I am also a believer in moderation where the sun is concerned. Get a reasonable amount of sunlight, but at times choose the shady side of the road, or wear a protective covering for your head. In some cases, too much sun has attacked the nose, creating tiny pimples which could be symptoms of something more serious— probably cancer.

I do not go in for conscious breathing when walking. You will find, if you do a lot of it, that you will naturally breathe more, and that your body will become thoroughly oxygenated. If, however, you are going uphill, it might be helpful to add a little in the way of breathing. In this respect, I would like to quote Dr. Francis W. Palfrey, who in the *New England Journal of Medicine* (246: 826, 1952) noted that the Swiss mountain guide walks all day at the same rate and rhythm without apparent fatigue. He also noticed that "with an increase in the grade ascended, the guide also shortens the step, perhaps to only a few inches in length.

[203]

It is a matter of shifting into low gear to prevent the engine from laboring."

Up to a very short time ago the general trend of thought in medical practice regarding reducing weight was to depend entirely on cutting down the amount of food. Exercise? Limit it to a rapid movement of the head from left to right when the strawberry shortcake is passed. Medical literature is full of condemnatory statements regarding the place of exercise in weight-reducing regimens.

The most ridiculous statement I ever saw in a magazine was the following: "Professor Arthur Steinhaus of George Williams College in Chicago reported that although exercise is important to general well-being, it is highly overrated as an aid to persons who want to reduce. To lose a pound, he reported, an average man weighing 155 pounds would have to do one of the following things: wrestle for $5\frac{1}{2}$ hours; fence for eight hours; saw wood for $10\frac{1}{2}$ hours; play ping pong for $17\frac{1}{4}$ hours; play billiards for $32\frac{1}{2}$ hours; walk 144 miles at the rate of two miles an hour; run 100 yards in 10 seconds 129 times; or climb the 555-foot Washington Monument 48 times."

It depends on *what* you have eaten as to how much you will lose in subsequent exercise. A meal heavy with bananas and fruit which contains a lot of water will just melt off with a little exercise. Meat and bread are harder to get off. It also depends at what stage you're in in your reducing program. Recently acquired fat, for instance, will come off very nicely with exercise.

There can be no question that the bulk of weight reduction must come from a lessened consumption of

[204]

food. Exercise, in a reducing program, must be used for a different purpose. To describe what I mean, I would like to quote a statement made by a physician who throws a different light on the value of exercising. He said, "Exercise has a useful place if the patient clearly understands that it contributes little to weight reduction per se, but that it serves other purposes, such as improved physical well-being and muscle tone."

In *Better Health* (Spring, 1951) it is expressed this way: "All they care about is losing weight according to the scale, when actually, all they should be caring about is losing dimensions in their hips, waist, bust, neck and thighs.

"Muscle weighs more than fat. If a woman happens to be the active big-bones type, with well-developed muscle, she might very well lose little weight in pounds, because her muscle gives her weight, but she'd be losing flesh and getting smaller in her dimensions."

To lose much in the way of dimension in the body, it means that there must be exercise as well as reduction in food, because exercise causes a compaction of the tissues (an increase in the specific gravity of the body). To a heart case this is most important, because if the specific gravity is low, due to lack of exercise (that is, if the body's tissues are not dense or compact), there is a retention of nitrogen compounds in the blood which causes imbalances in it. No blood imbalance is good for the heart. Where the body is compactly built, it can operate more efficiently with less strain upon the heart.

People say to me, "Isn't it boring to walk by yourself for a whole hour?" My answer is, "No. It is not boring." To me walking time is thinking time. As I walk along

[205]

I observe what passes before me. I notice the architecture of the buildings; I study the faces of people, the sky, trees, birds, plants and so forth. Incidentally, it is good for the eyes to look at the distant landscape. It exercises eye muscles that people rarely use in their close daily work at home and in the office. That is why seamen have good eyesight. They scan the horizon so much.

But walking with a companion makes the time go three times as fast. I would like to suggest walking conferences on the part of business people—but no stopping in at bars or for a soft drink. The coffee break is a vicious American habit. Dr. Frederick C. Swartz, at a conference at the University of Michigan, said that if you want to avoid shaky hands and a tottering gait in later life, give up your coffee break for a brief walk. He stated that "physical exercise begun early in life and continued into the advanced years is capable of delaying the physical stigma of aging and prolonging life expectancy as much as 8 to 10 years." And in my opinion the older you get, the more you should walk. I heard of a 115-year-old man who used to walk gently on and off all day long. That's for me when I'm 115. This man must have been all bone and muscle—in other words, possessed of a very high specific gravity.

In the city of Berkeley Heights, N.J., when the question came up of spending $30,000 for additional school buses, the town built walking paths for the pupils instead. It is working out very well. Every city and town should provide similar walking paths for young and old, and encourage hiking clubs. There should be a national back-to-the-walk movement.

DeQuincey once said about Wordsworth: "I calculate that with these identical legs Wordsworth must have traversed a distance of 180,000 English miles, a mode of exertion to which he was indebted for a life of unclouded happiness, and we for much of what is excellent in his writings." Wordsworth lived to 80 in a time when people died very young.

In my own case I have used my walks at times to figure out plots for plays and stories. When I find myself in a tight spot in working on a play, out I go for a walk, and the thoughts then begin to flow beautifully.

If you walk a lot, you will become a happier as well as healthier person. There is a great physical reaction in it that you feel as a gentle purring. It is a remarkable tonic for the nervous system. Unhappy people who go to psychiatrists should try walking. It is far better medicine for the sick of mind and for those with sick hearts. Walking is as important as food.

A little more attention to what some researchers call "the second heart" would take a lot of people off pills and keep them out of hospitals. Nature has provided our busy hearts with an auxiliary system to ease the load of pushing some 72,000 quarts of blood through the system every 24 hours, over nearly 100,000 miles of circulatory "roads." The help comes from the muscles in the feet, calves, thighs, buttocks and abdomen. As they work they rhythmically contract and release, squeezing the veins, forcing the blood along. It's nature's way of moving the blood to the heart and brain in spite of gravity.

The key to the efficiency of this system is walking. Walking makes the muscles below the abdomen do

[207]

their part in helping the heart. Without the push from these muscles, the blood tends to pool in the belly and in the feet. The heart has to pitch in with more and bigger beats to move that blood delivering essential nutrition to the tissues and flushing dangerous wastes.

Man is unique in his need for a "second heart." In four-legged animals, the circulation doesn't have much of a struggle against gravity because all the vital organs are on the same level; the heart, the brain, the lungs and even the reproductive glands have an easy time getting all the blood they need. But man stands up! Nature had to devise a way to pump the blood straight up, and the muscles around the veins were pressed into service. They work best when we walk.

All of this explains a lot about why walking has become so important in the treatment of heart patients. Doctors know now that it's the best way to make the muscles to take over their share of the work and relieve a damaged heart. Even a little walk improves circulation, and it costs the heart nothing. In truth, say authors Aaron Sussman and Ruth Goode, in *The Magic of Walking* (Simon and Schuster, New York), people whose heart rate and blood pressure are high, will find that a regimen of regular walking—not necessarily far or fast—brings the heart rate and blood pressure down to normal levels.

The "second heart" system worked like a charm for half a million years, then a lot of us stopped walking. No need anymore for walking to hunt; then no need for walking to farm. Now we no longer even walk to our jobs. If people are getting more heart disease, more digestive and elimination problems and more flabby

[208]

muscles than ever before, a good share of the blame is surely due to physical inactivity.

Surgeons prescribe walking a few steps within hours after an operation. This hospital procedure, which began originally as a measure against blood clots forming in patients kept inactive too long, showed its value in other unexpected ways—more rapid circulation, faster healing, improved muscle tone, better digestion and elimination. Patients forced to get out of bed and on their feet, no matter how painful it seems, feel a boost in morale. How sick can you be if you can stand up and move around on your own?

Walk More, Weigh Less

If people would walk more they would probably weigh less. Not that walking is the quickest way to chop off a fast 20 pounds. It isn't. But regular walking can keep your weight at the proper level. If you put yourself on an easy, daily walking schedule at the first sign of an unwanted pound, you have an excellent chance of holding your own in the eternal battle of the beltline.

A walk can skim the fat off the top of your calorie day. An hour's worth of walking uses up about 300 calories, and these are the few extra calories that pack themselves into wide waistlines, unflattering hips and multiple chins. As Sussman and Goode point out, nobody gains weight suddenly. It's just the discovery that's sudden—and painful. If you gain a fifth of a pound a week you may not notice it until the end of a year when the fifths have piled up into ten pounds.

[209]

So many of us gain weight after 35, because our activities lessen and we don't realize it. As a man gets older, he becomes more successful. He moves from the old two-story to a ranch house or even a fashionable apartment. And there go the stairs. He can afford a second car so walking to the bus stop is out. His executive job no longer calls for trotting around the plant; he sits behind a desk. Economic progress is costing him a healthy heart.

Back home after a tension-filled day, he heads for a snack and a drink (both heavy on calories) to help him relax. A brisk walk would do it better. More than that, the walk eliminates drinking time and takes off some of the excess calories accumulated during the day.

Overweight people hate to work at losing. They come up with this one: walking makes you hungry, makes you eat more, eventually makes you heavier than ever. To quote Dr. Jean Mayer, Harvard nutritionist, "If you don't walk at all, you may well become a little *less* hungry if you start walking for an hour a day. If you are already active increase your activity, your appetite will go up, but not so much that you won't profit from the activity."

If you're overweight, take a chance. Walking can't hurt you. On the whole habitual walkers tend to be moderate eaters; they rarely need a reducing diet; they run lean, not pudgy.

So walk for the help it gives your "second heart"; walk for an easy way to keep your weight under control; walk for how good it makes you feel and for the joy of a few private moments in the fresh air.

[210]

CHAPTER XXV

The Story of the Five Hills

J. I. Rodale

I have had an experience in connection with my daily walking program that is worth relating. As my readers know, for the last few years I have been walking, from an hour to two hours a day, with wonderful benefit to my physical condition especially with a reduction of my pulse from about 85 to about 65 to 72. But something occurred one winter which indicated to me that there is more to walking than just walking.

We had taken a house for the entire winter in Palm Beach so that I would be able to do my walking every day. But it did not work out the way I expected. I did my regular stint of walking every day but somehow I did not feel that I was thriving on it as well as I did at home. For one thing, my speaking voice became weaker. I didn't have my blood pressure taken while there, but when we came home and I had it checked I found that it had jumped from 120 to about 140.

Well, this called for some thinking, but for the time being nothing came of it. About a month later I had my blood pressure taken again, but this time it had gone back to normal, namely 120. And my voice had come back to its normal pitch. You can believe that I immediately set myself to do some tall thinking. It did not take me long to get what I believe to be the answer for what had happened in Florida.

Palm Beach is as flat as a pancake, whereas at home I walked among gently rolling hills. The effort of pushing upward while walking evidently has much more beneficial effect than walking on the flat. Besides, at home I slept on the second floor, and went up and down stairs many times a day. In Palm Beach our rented house was a one-story affair.

So, I realized at once that walking up hill is far more healthful than walking on a flat surface. It so happens that there are some steep hills near our farm, which I had been avoiding. Now I began to lay out a daily walk of one hour that took in only the steepest hills I could find. These are really hills! One of them is almost like a sheer wall. The effect? Amazing! And me a heart case that was turned down for life insurance in 1953 (Metropolitan Life Insurance Co.).

I took these hills with a confidence engendered by taking large protective doses of vitamin E (1,200 milligrams daily of mixed tocopherols). I am so delighted with what this hill-walking has done for me that if ever

[212]

we choose a name for our farm it will be *The Five Hills Organic Farm.*

From this point on I became hill-conscious, talking about hill-walking at every opportunity. One man said, "I think you've got something, Mr. Rodale. So many of the prime ministers of England have been Scotchmen, who came from very hilly regions. Evidently hill-walking develops the mind as well as the body." Could this account for Scotch geniuses like Sir Walter Scott, Robert Burns, and many others? The Scotch seem to be a vigorous, strong-minded, mentally alert race. In the case of Jenny Geddes, who in church threw a stool at a reformer because she disagreed with his views, was her character molded by a lifetime of walking in steep hills? It is a noteworthy fact that races that live in these regions are aware that they "need" these hills. When the Scotch or Welsh emigrate to the United States they always choose hilly regions for their colonies.

I met an old man who still remembered a doctor of his youth in New York City, who made all his patients walk 20 hills. In those days the main disease was called auto-intoxication (which had nothing to do with autos). This doctor with his 20-hill regimen effected sensational cures.

One man of about 55 whom I spoke to told me an amazing thing. It seems that he was suffering from a sexual condition. At the end of intercourse he would experience a sharp pain. After about 3 weeks of hill walking he no longer experienced such pains.

I was recently reading *The Citadel* by A. J. Cronin, and came to an interesting passage. A woman is be-

[213]

rating a doctor who seldom prescribed medicines. She says, "Go on with you, Doctor. He's reg'lar quee-ar. Mostly he don't give medicine at all. Why when Megan Rhys Morgan, what's had to have medicine all her life, went to him, he told her to walk two mile up the mountain every day and stop boggin' herself with hog-wash" (meaning medicine). More physicians should suggest hill walking to their patients and they will dispense less medicine.

Thomas Hobbes, an English writer and philosopher who lived for 91 years and whose last book was published when he was 87, is thus described in *Brief Lives* by John Aubrey (1625-1697), who knew him during the last half of the philosopher's life:

"In the countrey, for want of a tennis-court, he would walke uphill and downe-hill in the parke, till he was in a great sweat, and then give the servant some money to rubbe him . . . at night, when he was abed, and the dores made fast, and was sure nobody heard him, he sang aloud (not that he had a very good voice) for his health sake; he did believe it did his Lunges good, and conduced much to prolong his life."

We are told that in Bulgaria and Yugoslavia there are sections where people live to be very old. Usually the reason is given that these people drink a certain kind of sour milk that teems with beneficial microscopic organisms. I wonder if these people live in mountainous regions and have hardened their bodies by walking daily in steep hills. Perhaps it is the effect of both. However, it would be a good thing if some research organization compared the death rates and

[214]

the extent of chronic disease as between hilly and flat regions.

When I began to walk my five hills I took it easy at first because of my heart condition. I would stop to rest for 20 or 30 seconds whenever I felt too tired to go on with comfort. At the beginning I would have to stop 10 times before reaching the top of a hill. On the first day I had to go to bed for 3 hours after I returned from the walk—I was so fatigued. Within two days I did not require any nap at all. In fact, on one of these days I experienced a wonderful feeling of euphoria which I had not felt in a long time . . . a strange, pleasant exhilaration.

Gradually I was able to go higher on a hill before making my first stop. I figured that by the end of the summer I would be able to make all the hills without any stops at all. But I was able to accomplish this by June 28, approximately a month and a half after I began my hill-walking regimen.

The first time that I made the longest hill without stopping, I must have been helped along by some church singing that came out of the Salisbury Church that is located at the top. It seemed to be inspired with a divine fire. They were singing "O Living Bread from Heaven." I stood transfixed, drinking it in with tremendous enjoyment. If you wish to experience a heavenly feeling, walk up a long hill and suddenly come upon a church at the top with singing voices coming forth. It takes physical heights to lead to spiritual heights. Moses walked up to Mt. Sinai to get the Ten Commandments. Christ walked up to the mount to

[215]

give His famous sermon. Walking hills will lift you up in more senses than one.

One particular week-day I walked up this hill and the church of course was empty, but the door being invitingly open, I went in. What a wonderful feeling surged over me. Oh, how I wished a minister was there that I could communicate my feelings to him. Churches should be on top of hills and the people should walk up to worship. Please excuse me for being carried away from the main theme of my subject.

During the first month of this hill-walking period my weight was coming down from over 170 to 162. One hundred and sixty-two is a magic figure in the functioning of my body. I have found this to be so several times before. Evidently my frame and heart were designed to work with not over 162 pounds, and the minute I get over that weight I can feel it. When I got down to 162 it seemed I could make the hills with greater ease.

It has been said that walking stairs takes about 10 times the energy of walking on the flat. Exactly how much more energy it takes to walk up a hill depends, of course, on the extent of the grade, but based on the pulling of my muscles as I climbed, I know that it not only takes much more energy, but it uses more muscles and uses them harder. I also know that it causes the glands of the body to be more active and to produce their secretions to a greater extent. On a steep hill I could feel the pull on the muscles of my entire mid-region, and in the back of my legs, near the thighs. Exercise is known to build new capillaries, so I imagine

[216]

that hill-walking must be very effective in this direction. It probably builds collateral circulation facilities like mad. This assures sufficient channels to carry the blood to and from the heart. It is like the construction of additional streets in a city. Hill-walking also greatly dilates the blood vessels, thus stimulating the blood circulation.

I know that in walking hills the main pull is in the mid-region where the small and large intestines, the stomach, the liver, kidneys, pancreas, spleen and the reproductive organs are located. Thus, all of these organs benefit.

We must not overlook the fact also that when you walk up a hill you must also walk down, and from my experience even walking downward on a steep grade takes more energy than walking on the flat. In Europe they used to run races down steep hills and the Yugoslavians always won. Evidently, their country is so hilly that they have the means at hand to practice. As I said before, this could be the reason why there are so many old persons in Yugoslavia.

According to the newspapers I see where an 88-year-old Scotch lady who has lived in Yugoslavia for about 40 years is going to climb the Triglav peak, which is the highest mountain in that country. Last year she spent 14 hours climbing that mountain and afterwards said she felt very good. She uses a very slow walking pace. In another year or two I intend to go in for mountain walking, although I have no desire to go too high.

While in Germany recently, a friend told me about a doctor who was suffering from high blood pressure. He cured himself by walking to the top of mountains with the aid of two long sticks. Now he says, "I have 4 feet." He has so conditioned himself that he can out-climb far younger persons.

Another friend told me about a sanatorium in Bad Nannheim, which specializes in heart cases. It makes use of 3 long hills, one with a 5 per cent grade, the second with a 10 per cent grade, and the third with a grade of 15 per cent. The patient first slowly walks on the 5 per cent grade hill, accompanied by a nurse, resting frequently, and sitting on benches to look at the beautiful view of the valley. Gradually, as he becomes hardened, he is able to climb the 15 per cent hill without resting, and with a great strengthening of his heart. This has been a standard method in that sanatorium for over a hundred years.

Now, coming to the direct results I obtained from my hill-walking. Within a short time I noticed better bowel movements, I felt a definite improvement on my lung action, I could breathe easier, I seemed to have more energy and noticed an improvement in my spirits, although I don't usually suffer from depression. Now I sleep better and have a greater capacity for mental work. I am able to eat bread without heart symptoms developing. One of the most unusual results is the ability to get out of bed with less sleeping lameness in my side. Usually this completely dissipates moments after I arise, but now I get very little if any of it. I believe that this condition is due to a slight rupture that I have had since 1922, but which doesn't trouble me.

[218]

When I used to turn over in sleep I felt this slight lameness, but after hill-walking I can turn over in bed without the least pain. One of the most significant results is that even on the hottest day, the under-arm perspiration arising from a hill walk has no odor. Incidentally, don't let anyone tell you that you can't lose weight in summer by exercising. Walking hills on a hot day just laps the weight off. Use the summertime for losing weight, and the winter for maintaining it. But don't take salt. If you do, you will want to drink water, which will restore all the weight you have lost.

If you are deciding on a vacation spot pick out a hilly region. If you wish to move to a new location, choose a hilly one. Your children will grow up healthier there. It would be interesting to make juvenile delinquency surveys as between hilly and flat regions. Athletes, pugilists, etc. can condition themselves by doing hill-walking.

Today, as I walk my five hills, I have a terrific undercurrent of a feeling that this hill-walking is doing wonders for my general health. So, this psychosomatic dimension must be added to the values of these walks, for it helps as well as the physical effect.

I have a Battle Creek walking machine which I will use at home during the freezing and snowy weather of winter. On it one walks at a grade, similar to walking uphill. This winter I do not expect to go to Florida, and if I take a vacation in some warm climate for a few weeks or so, I shall choose some hilly, tropical country. Experience is the greatest teacher.

[219]

CHAPTER XXVI

Can Exercise be Harmful?

J. I. Rodale

Is it dangerous for a heart case to exercise? To answer this question we must first analyze what is included in exercise. I think common sense would dictate that we should eliminate its more strenuous forms, such as tennis, basketball, etc. In our discussion we will include for our purposes such exercises as walking, golf, horseback riding, setting-up exercises, etc. To answer the question in the first sentence on this basis, I would say that 99 per cent of heart cases can safely exercise.

It used to be thought that the average heart attack came in the throes of severe activity, but recent studies indicate that this is not so. *Time,* of October 19, 1953, throws some light on the subject:

"Coronary patients who think they can stave off

further attacks by unnatural idleness are mistaken,"
said Manhattan's Dr. Arthur M. Master. "Of 2,200
heart attacks, he found 23 per cent occurred during
sleep, 29 per cent while at work, 24 per cent during
mild activity, 13 per cent during walking at an ordinary pace, 9 per cent during moderate activity and
only 2 per cent during unusual exertion."

Dr. Master found that "the percentage of attacks
that occurred during sleep, rest, mild, moderate or severe activity coincided with the proportion of the day
usually spent in these states. The occurrence of coronary occlusion thus seems to be coincidental with what
the sufferer is doing when the attack occurs," Dr.
Master said.

The following is a letter that Dr. G. C. Willcocks
sent to the *Medical Journal of Australia* and which
was printed in the August 14, 1954 issue:

"Sir . . . Recently 100 consecutive cases of acute
coronary occlusion at Sydney Hospital were investigated with regard to the relationship to exertion. Of
these 100, 10 were in bed at the onset, 15 were at rest,
five were in the street, five were at work (nature not
stated), five were walking (one up a steep hill and one
up steps), one was bicycling, one coughing, two were
in doctors' rooms, one sweeping, and one picking up a
hat. In 10 the onset was gradual with angina of increasing severity. In the remainder, the patient's occupation at the time of onset was not stated. Thus, out
of 55 patients in whom the occupation at the time of
onset of coronary occlusion was ascertained, three may
have been undergoing a considerable degree of exer-

tion (one bicycling, one walking up a steep hill and one walking up steps). As to those who were said to be working at the time of onset, there was no indication as to the type of work.

"This series shows that 55 persons suffering from coronary atheroma (for atheroma causes 90 per cent of coronary lesions) had been going about their daily life for months or years, without any ill effects, except angina in some. All these persons must have been exerting themselves for years or months in the ordinary course of their lives, because they did not feel ill and had no reason to be restrained in their exertions. It would be no exaggeration to say that in this series of 55 persons, there would be thousands of exertions in the course of a few months, and only three of the patients sustained an occlusion at a time of exertion.

"The above seems to indicate that exertion plays little part in the onset of an acute coronary occlusion."

On page 1264 (April 2, 1955) of the *Journal of the American Medical Association* appears the statement: "Stout thus summarizes the matter: 'The mass of evidence indicates that work and exercise do not precipitate coronary thrombosis, coronary occlusion, or myocardial infarction.' " All three are forms of heart attacks.

Thus, we have shown that it is not exercise that is the cause of a heart attack. Now I would like to show, on the other hand, that exercise is a form of insurance to prevent a heart attack. In this respect I would like to consider a series of studies that were made in London, the results of which appeared in *The Lancet* for

[222]

November 21 and 28, 1953, under the title "Coronary Heart Disease and Physical Activity of Work." The occurrence of coronary heart disease was studied in drivers and conductors of buses, trams and trolley buses, in motormen and guards on subways, a group comprising 31,000 men between the ages of 35 and 64.

Peculiarly it showed that "coronary heart disease behaves differently in the drivers and in the conductors . . . the immediate deaths accounted for 31 per cent in the drivers as against 19 per cent in the conductors.

"Is this a chance phenomenon? . . . the greater physical activity of 'conducting' (on these double-decker vehicles) is a cause of the lower incidence and mortality in the conductors . . . the underground railwaymen had a pattern of disease similar to that of the road vehicle drivers . . . the physical in the conductors' work may be a protective factor, safeguarding them in middle age from some of the worst manifestations of coronary heart disease suffered by less active workers."

The group of investigators then began a study of Post Office and Civil Service workers to see if the results would parallel those of the transport workers. Quoting from the report, "There is no doubt that the physical exertion at work of the postman is greater than that of any of the other grades included, and there are three truly sedentary grades for comparison— telephonists, executives and clerks. . . . The results show that the total incidence of coronary heart diseases is lower in the postmen than in the sedentary grades . . . . the experience of the postal workers and Civil

[223]

Servants may therefore be said to resemble that of the transport workers; the physically active group (the postmen) have rather less coronary heart disease; and what disease they do have is less severe . . . the main interest of these findings in postal workers and Civil Servants lies in the support they provide for the idea suggested by the observation of the transport workers —that physical activity at work is important in relation to the coronary heart disease of middle-aged men . . .

"The present postulate may thus be extended to include all coronary deaths: 'That men doing physically active work have a lower mortality from coronary heart disease in middle age than men in less active work.' "

A third study was made along the same lines and I will quote from the report in regard to it: "A group of light occupations which are highly specialized and require considerable skill and training was isolated from social class III in the Registrar-General's occupational mortality data. Such occupations are potter, compositor, French polisher, railway engine driver, railway signalman, and the police. . . . The mortality from coronary heart disease in this special group of light occupations was found to be substantially greater than in the heavy workers of social class III, and this excess was apparent from 45-54 through 70-74 years of age."

An article in the *British Journal of Industrial Medicine* (10: 245, 1953) by doctors Morris and Heady also discusses a study which revealed that deaths from

[224]

coronary heart disease "in middle age may be less common among men engaged in physically active work than among those in sedentary jobs. . . . It was found that the mortality from coronary heart disease at 45 to 64 years of age among the heavy workers was rather less than half that of the light workers." Incidentally in this survey it was found that there were six other conditions in which there was greater mortality among middle-aged men engaged in lighter work. These were cancer of the lung, appendicitis, diseases of the prostate, duodenal ulcer, diabetes and cirrhosis of the liver.

In commenting on this article the *Canadian Medical Association Journal* (February, 1954) says: "That there may be a 'general factor' of health and disease associated with physical effort and sedentariness in work. . . . Physical work may be 'a way of life' conducive to good health."

The fact that inactivity may be harmful to the body is illustrated in the case of penned-up chickens. Here is an item from *Science Digest* of March, 1952, quoting from an article in *Modern Medicine*. "More than 70 per cent of chickens one year of age or more have evidence of spontaneous arteriosclerosis of the arteries of the heart. The sclerosis is shown more by connective tissue proliferation of the arterial wall than by fatty deposits."

As a "gentleman" farmer I have seen the difference in health between chickens who can roam about the barnyard and those who are cooped up.

In the last few years medical opinion has veered towards "work" for heart cases, after a heart attack.

[225]

The following is a summary of findings discussed at a special symposium on rehabilitation of heart cases, held in Cincinnati, Oct. 29, 1956, as printed in the *New York Times* the next day:

"Most industrial jobs have low energy requirements. Housewives work harder than do men at plants or offices in most cases. A cardiac's heart does not have to work harder to perform given tasks than does the heart of a normal individual. Many patients make surprising improvements after they return to work. Under-exertion may be more of a hazard for heart patients than overexertion. Psychological damage may be greater than physiological damage following a heart ailment. Physicians should not be afraid to advise heart patients to exercise and work."

The question may naturally arise whether there are certain kinds of heart conditions where caution should be the rule on the question of exercise. There are a few. One case, of an enlarged and feeble heart, could walk only 6 steps before he had to stop on account of pain and exhaustion. Such a person should not exercise. In this case, an operation was performed on the heart, and at present this man can get around easily and even climb stairs.

In cases of rupture of the myocardium (the muscular substance of the heart), exertion is especially risky. Where there has been some kind of incident in connection with the heart, conservatism would call for prudence in connection with exercise. In such cases the physician will usually advise the proper course. Dr. U. L. Brown, in the *Medical Journal of Australia*,

[226]

February 13, 1954, gives some good advice in this respect. He says: "Every case must be individually assessed, and you must steadily avoid the far too common and equally ignorant assertion that the manifestation of coronary disease marks the end of a man's useful working life. . . . A man may do in safety anything he can do in comfort, and he is well advised to remain active within his limits of comfortable exertion, rather than sink into himself and lead a life of invalidism. If he remains active, I believe that the development of the collateral circulation is assisted by the increased blood flow which accompanies effort, whereas it is probably hindered by the stagnating blood flow of ill-advised rest."

Here is some advice by Dr. Joseph B. Wolffe, given in the *N.Y. State Journal of Medicine,* Aug. 1, 1956. He says, "Sustained, judicious physical activity over a lifetime seems to be a prophylactic and therapeutic measure in atherogenesis (a form of hardening of the arteries). Mild, temporary anoxia (oxygen deficiency) resulting from indicated physical exercise might reasonably be the best vasodilator (causing a widening of the blood vessels). Noncompetitive recreational activities are to be preferred with emphasis on play rather than display. However, sudden unaccustomed strenuous activity should be stringently avoided. Whenever possible, productive work should be continued."

CHAPTER XXVII

Jog Your Way to Better Health

Benjamin Franklin all his life loved to swim. He lived happily and usefully into his 85th year. The two facts may well have some connection.

There are those who deny the need of the average person for regular and vigorous exercise. But the consensus of those who should know seems to be that most of us are much better off if we adopt a regimen which demands a reasonable amount of physical activity beyond what is required in getting to and from our cars.

"Concurrent with a reduction in the requirements for physical activity in modern living, there has been an increase in death and disability from cardiovascular diseases associated with 'athero-thrombotic' processes. . . . Although we do not consider a causal relationship

[228]

established, some excellent studies suggest that physical inactivity may be one of possibly many factors involved in the increasing prominence of ischemic vascular disease, the most significant form of which is coronary heart disease." So say Samuel M. Fox, III, M.D. and James S. Skinner, Ph.D., in an article, "Physical Activity and Cardiovascular Health" (*American Journal of Cardiology,* December, 1964).

The same authors also quote William Stokes, who in 1854 wrote concerning the "treatment of fatty degeneration of the heart":

"In the present state of our knowledge, the adoption of the following principles . . . the management of a case of incipient fatty disease seems justifiable . . . he must adopt early hours, and pursue a system of graduated muscular exercise; and, it will often happen that after perseverance in this system, the patient will be enabled to take an amount of exercise with pleasure and advantage which at first was totally impossible. . . . This treatment by muscular exercise is obviously more proper in younger persons than in those advanced in life. The symptoms of debility of the heart are often removable by a regulated course of gymnastics, or by pedestrian exercise."

Doctors Fox and Skinner tell about a great deal of recent research in more than 200 hospitals and hospital groups. One finding: "Physical activity of work is a protection against coronary (ischemic) heart disease. Men in physically active jobs have less coronary heart disease during middle age, and what disease they have is less severe, and they develop it later than men in

[229]

YOUR DIET AND YOUR HEART

physically inactive jobs." A further conclusion: "Regular physical exercise could be one of the 'ways of life' that promote health in middle age, and ischemic heart disease may be in some degree a deprivation syndrome, a deficiency disease."

One answer that a million or so men have already found is jogging. You know what jogging is. When you used to be a boy scout, it was called Scout's Pace in your handbook. You run away and as soon as you begin to feel a little tired or breathless, you slow down to a walk and keep moving while you're resting. As soon as you've had a chance to get your breath back, you start running again.

Working out in this simple fashion, you can go an incredibly long way without overtiring yourself. But is it good exercise? Well, according to Major Kenneth Cooper of the U.S. Air Force Medical Corps Fitness Program, it is not only good exercise—it is the best exercise in the world. Extensive tests have been made at the Lackland Air Base in the development of a program to keep pilots in top health.

It has been established that out of dozens of ways to use the body vigorously, the very top way of using up energy, burning up calories and spreading life-giving oxygen throughout the tissues is running. And jogging is the best way known to run and keep on running far beyond what your normal capacity could be expected to be, and still not overstrain yourself in any way.

Here is Dr. Cooper's surprising list of physical conditioning activities in order of their effectiveness: 1. running or jogging; 2. swimming; 3. cycling; 4. walking; 5. stationary running (running in place); 6. handball; 7. basketball; 8. squash. They are all good exercises, but jogging, which is at the head of the list, is also the easiest and the safest for everyone.

Where can you jog? You can do it anywhere. A few years ago it might have looked silly to see a man in a sweatshirt running through the streets of a city. But by now so many people have taken up jogging that it has become a common sight, and people hardly notice any more. When they do notice, it is with admiration for someone they know is taking the right measures to keep or improve his physical fitness and stay healthy all his life.

Nor do you have to jog alone. Jogging clubs have sprung up in every major city of the United States as well as many small cities and towns. A phone call to your local YMCA is probably all it will take for you to locate such a club. If you can't find one or don't like clubs, how about taking your wife out for a jog? It's as good for women as it is for men, and the women, since they are more figure conscious, get even more enthusiastic about the exercise once they are introduced to it. Track coach William J. Bowerman lists the following advantages to jogging, all of which will appeal to your wife:

1. Jogging improves the legs, making them slimmer and firmer. It trims the ankles and makes calves shapely.

2. It slims the waistline. It doesn't necessarily take off weight—it might even put some on the under-

[231]

weight. But in every case, the weight is redistributed and the waist gets slimmer.

3. It reduces the hips and flattens the abdomen.

4. Jogging firms sagging muscles all over the body. Even double chins and the upper arms somehow get exercise during jogging and firm up.

5. Finally, jogging doesn't cost anything and thus appeals to many thrifty housewives who might object even to the enrollment fee at a gym.

Here are some tips on jogging form that will help you get the greatest benefits from the exercise and experience the least discomfort.

Posture. Stand up straight while running and walking. This does not mean a military brace, but it does mean that you keep your head up and your back as straight as you naturally and comfortably can.

Arm movements. Keep your elbows bent and slightly away from the body, letting them move rhythmically forward and back.

Leg movement. Move your legs from the hips with an easy, unforced action. Lift from the knees keeping your ankles relaxed. Don't reach out for a long stride but let each step take you just a normally comfortable distance.

Breathing. Breathe through your mouth as well as your nose. Inhale as much air as possible. Getting that oxygen into your system is practically the name of the game.

Footstrike. Heel to toe is preferred. You land on your heel and roll forward onto your toe before that leg takes off again. It is least tiring over long distances and

[232]

JOG YOUR WAY TO BETTER HEALTH

causes the least strain. However, if you don't find this particular way of striking the foot comfortable, don't stop on that account. Let your own comfort be your basic guide.

You should jog at least three times a week for half an hour each time. Once you get started, however, you're going to find that you have so much fun jogging and it makes you feel so good that you may do it every day or you may do it for longer periods of time. That's up to you. But take the half hour at a time three times a week as your minimum, and you can be sure you are going to stay in reasonably good condition all the days of your life.

CHAPTER XXVIII

Exercise the Easy Way

Have you tried exercising while you're sitting in your office?—or rocking on the back porch?—or while you're sitting watching TV? You can and you should! Too many people think exercise must start with a closetful of new equipment ranging from golf clubs to dumbbells and a rowing machine. The very idea of all of this extra expense and effort defeats them. If this is exercise, they'll skip it.

Exercise, however, can be what you want it to be, costly or free, strenuous or mild. The important thing is to get *some* form of exercise, because the body needs it as surely as it needs nutrition, if it is to maintain itself properly.

Exercise Good for Weak Hearts

The relationship between the healthy heart and exercise is well established. The *Journal of the American*

Medical Association (December 17, 1960) puts it this
way: "As a general rule, people engaged in occupations requiring regular and vigorous exercise have a
lower incidence of coronary thrombosis than people
doing sedentary work. . . ."

Paul Dudley White, M.D., famous heart specialist,
was more explicit and emphatic about the value of
exercise to the health of the heart and the rest of the
body, in a pamphlet edited by him entitled *Exercise
Is Good Preventive Medicine.* "Exercise is important
for everybody, whether they've been sick or not. Of
course a person in an acute illness, whether it's from
heart disease, or pneumonia or any other kind of illness,
has got to be treated for that immediate disease. But,
after recovery, graded exercise can favor the progress
of convalescence and rehabilitation.

"There are immediate physical effects of exercise on
the circulation of the blood. Good muscle tone in the
arms and particularly in the legs, resulting from regular exercise, maintains an improved circulation of blood
in the veins. . . .

"In addition to its beneficial effect on skeletal muscle tone, exercise also improves the tone of the diaphragm, which results in better function as the piston
of a pump, not only to bring a full supply of oxygen to
the lungs with removal of carbon dioxide, but also to
suction blood into the heart. . . ."

Doctor White goes on to say, "Digestion, when meals
follow exercise and do not just precede it, and bowel
function are improved by exercise. Not infrequently
vigorous sport renders laxative medicine quite unneces-

[235]

sary. Sleep is favored, too, in fact, a brisk long walk in the evening may be more helpful as a hypnotic than any medicine, highball or television show.

"It matters little, if at all, what type of exercise it is, provided it suits the strength and liking of the individual concerned. It is well to establish a regular habit and to maintain it through thick and thin. One should regard it as just as essential to good health as eating, sleeping and working."

So says an expert on heart disease, who recognizes the value of exercise in every aspect of good health. But notice what Dr. White has to say about the *type* of exercise for the best results: any kind! We agree. Any kind of exercise at all is infinitely better than no kind. So you have perfect freedom to please yourself.

There aren't many of us who feel inclined to run 3 times around the block each morning or do a hundred push-ups before breakfast. For those who have trained for it, and are used to strenuous effort, this kind of exercise is a fine way to keep your vigor. But you can't start out like that at 50, and expect a soft body to respond without complaint. What then—forget exercise? Of course not. But take the easy way out until you're ready for bigger things. Remember, the important thing is to do *something,* and do it regularly.

For an opener, we have yet to see easier, or more worthwhile exercises than those proposed by Karen Roon for a lady's magazine a few years ago. They are designed to relieve tension, and you needn't stir from your easy chair for most of them.

Do you notice, when you take time to think of it,

[236]

that you hold your jaw set tight without really being
conscious of it? That's tension. An exercise that will
help to relieve that requires merely that you blow out,
lips pursed. Blow hard. Wait a moment, quietly. If
you feel like sighing, sigh; if you want to yawn, yawn.
Your jaw will drop and your whole chest expand.
Enjoy it—that's relaxation.

If you have a habit of clenching your teeth uncon-
sciously, place your index fingers on the side of your
face in front of your ears, and lightly rotate the muscles
you feel for a few seconds. (You'll find it easy to locate
the proper spot by feel.) Do this morning and evening.
Then follow up by repeatedly dropping the jaw. Let
your jaw relax.

Think about your shoulders. Do they feel tense? Try
shoulder rolling to make shoulders and upper chest
flexible, and restore good breathing. Then pull the
shoulders forward, down, and up again while exhaling.
Now reverse the movement by swinging back when
you exhale.

If your neck tends to get stiff, sit up straight, drop
your head so the chin nearly touches the chest. The
lower jaw hangs loose. While inhaling through the
nose, start pulling the head to the right, not lifting the
shoulder. Keep swinging your head in a circle, holding
your breath until you complete the circle. Exhale; lift
your head; rest. Start over and do the other side the
same way.

For a quiet exercise for the eyes, lie down or sit.
Let the eyelids drop over the eyes without pressing
them together. Imagine your eyeballs to be dropping

[237]

out of their sockets, back into the skull. The feeling of empty eye sockets relaxes the eye muscles.

An exercise for keeping stiffness out of the arms consists merely of firmly massaging the area on the palm between the base of the thumb and base of the index finger. Then the massaging is repeated at the same location on the back of the hand. Now the other hand. The thumbs are then rotated in a wide circle.

If you're just feeling tired, sit comfortably in a hard chair. Put your feet flat on the floor, toes slightly pointed in. Put up heels and lower about 6 times. Inhale when you're pulling up, and exhale while lowering. Now raise and lower the toes in the same manner. Rest. Then do the movements alternately.

You can begin that easily. If you are consistent, you will benefit from these simple exercises. If you've been wondering what to do about tensions, pills are no answer, but these exercises are.

Suppose you're in bed, and have a minute before you must get up, or suppose you can't fall asleep at once. *McCall's* (January, 1958) offered some appealingly easy exercises you can do as you lie there.

1. To loosen up in general, lie flat on your back, with the left knee bent and the left foot flat. Now reach the right arm back and stretch the right leg out. Then repeat on the other side, alternating 10 times.

2. To relieve neck tension, lie on your back, knees bent and feet flat, with hands clasped behind your head. Then lift the left arm and shoulder reaching for the right hip with the left elbow. Relax, then switch sides and repeat 10 times.

[238]

3. For building chest and shoulder muscles, lie on your stomach, hands clasped behind your back. Now pull your shoulders and upper torso off the bed. Relax and do it again—ten times.

Here again, remember that the number of times suggested for each exercise is only a *suggestion*. You're the boss! If you like, do it only 8 times or 3 times—but do it!

A really fascinating mode of exercise, even if it does require that you get out of the arm chair to do it, is folk dancing. There are certainly few more pleasant ways to build yourself up. Consider the advantages: new social contacts, an interesting way to get the pure feeling of different culture, and a painless, graceful way to exercise that will give you enjoyment long after you have completed any formal instruction.

Most city recreation departments or high school evening instruction programs for adults include folk dancing classes. Few of them would be so exotic as the one offered by Sophia Delza to the interested personnel at the United Nations Building in New York. This lady teaches T'ai Chi Ch'yan, an ancient form of exercise which originated in China and "is intended to activate both the body and the mind," says *MD* magazine (September, 1961). The entire exercise is made up of 108 continuous rhythmic movements to various positions, each with some specific relationship to the other. "The essence of T'ai Chi Ch'yan is claimed to be the achievement of tranquility, not through any conscious effort but through the design and play within each movement."

[239]

That is the essence of our attitude toward a desirable exercise—a minimal conscious effort. Dancing certainly offers this, and folk dancing even more so, since the figures are so interesting and varied and a bit more active than the ballroom dancing most of us are used to doing, and it's all much more invigorating.

Doctors favor walking as a good, helpful and sensible exercise that will do something for anyone and can do no harm, except in the most unusual cases. One indication of the physical value of leg movement appeared in the *Archives of Surgery* (October, 1958). Doctors were anxious to find a means of keeping the patient "walking" during surgery. The leg muscles at rest tend to allow blood pools to form in the legs, and thus set the conditions considered most likely to allow the formation of blood clots. A method has been devised to stimulate the muscles in the calf of the leg during surgery so that they simulate walking conditions in the muscle structure, and cut down the possibility of circulatory trouble.

Obviously, walking is one method of keeping the circulation in good condition before a surgeon has to do it for you.

In the *Archives of Physical Medicine and Rehabilitation* (January, 1958), Dr. Gerald G. Hirschburg listed the following advantages of stairclimbing as an exercise: It requires 15 times as much energy to climb stairs as to walk on the level. This extra energy expenditure requires greater muscular effort, and this in turn constitutes a strengthening device. Stairclimbing may involve all of the muscles of the body, but has a

[240]

specific effect on the flexors and extensors of the trunk and legs.

Interestingly, in the process of stairclimbing, the exercise comes to the very muscles which are much less frequently used in the normal activities of ambulation. The flexor muscle of the foot, the hip and the abdominals are used when the foot is lifted to the next step. Level walking does not necessarily require muscular contraction against resistance. If the walker is lazy, he shuffles instead of lifting the feet; this can't happen when stairs are involved. They force one to take exercising steps.

(If you've walked yourself into a case of tired feet, you can handle that problem as you sit, too. Put your legs on a footstool, stretch and separate the toes as far as possible. Then grab with the toes, as though attempting to hold something tightly, for a few seconds. This bit of exercise will strengthen foot muscles and reduce fatigue.)

Automobiles are blamed, and rightly too, for eliminating many of our opportunities for exercise. But time spent in a car, either driving to work, or taking a trip, needn't be lost to exercise. Mr. John Compardo, a physical education instructor at an Allentown, Pennsylvania high school, reminded us forcefully of the great benefit to be derived from simple breathing exercises. They are good for everyone to do, and they can be done anywhere at any time—in a car, for example. Try these:

1. Take alternate deep inhalations and exhalations.

Try to suck in as much air as you can, and then when you exhale, make it last.

2. Inhale in short gulps or gasps until your lungs are full, then exhale in this identical putt-putt fashion.

3. This time don't try for a big air supply. Inhale and exhale in short, quick spasms. It will strengthen your diaphragm muscles.

4. Take a deep breath and hold it, stomach in, as you begin a tightening process of all the muscles from your toes to your scalp. It's easy to do. You can will the muscles to tense as you go from calf muscles, to thigh, stomach, back and chest muscles, then to neck, face, and scalp muscles. Relax and do it again several times.

For those who are willing to become more physical about the type of exercise they adopt, cycling comes highly recommended. *Scope Weekly* (November 6, 1957) quotes Dr. Harlan G. Metcalf, who headed the physical fitness drive in World War II, as saying it is the "perfect way to aid both physical and mental fitness." An eminent European doctor, says *Scope*, reports that cycling in the open air generally stops colds, that a "fast-moving, fully oxygenated blood stream obtained by pedal-pushing will not tolerate the cold germ."

Dr. Paul Dudley White lists a whole catalogue of health benefits through cycling:

1. It aids the circulation thereby making the heart's job easier, because the blood is actively moving in the legs.

2. The tone of the diaphragm is improved, thus aid-

ing the lungs in bringing in oxygen and pumping out carbon dioxide.

3. The brain is cleared.

4. The nerves are improved because cycling promotes good sleep.

5. Ulcers are avoided because digestion is aided by moderate cycling.

6. The weight is happily affected by the exercise cycling provides.

7. Cyclists should get a few extra years of life because many degenerative trends in the body are reversed or slowed down by this activity.

Swimming is another of those exercises which are universally endorsed by medical men. Every muscle is brought into play and the lung capacity is enlarged. All age groups can participate, each according to his own limitations. Swimming is also one of those easy, pleasant, but efficient methods of exercise, in which you are the boss in deciding how much you can take. When you stop enjoying it, stop doing it!

Make that your rule in the beginning. It's an encouraging thought, and one which will prevent your overdoing things. But be fair. Choose an exercise that you can and will do with some consistency. Even if you only do a little, you must remember to do it regularly. If you do, it will become easier and easier, and as your muscles and endurance build, you will want to do more and to do it longer. Start modestly, moderately, so that when you stop the day's effort, you will find yourself looking forward to what you can do tomorrow.

Longer life and health to enjoy it will be your reward.

[243]

CHAPTER XXIX

Better Hearts through Exercise

Despite the landmark achievements of medical research in perfecting open heart surgery, developing cardiovascular drugs, and creating artificial pumping devices, coronary heart disease still claims more lives than any other illness. Obesity, high cholesterol levels from whatever cause, heavy smoking, and a history of high blood pressure, all coupled with physical inactivity, appear to increase the risk of a heart attack by diminishing the amount of blood that flows through the arteries to the heart. Yet, it is becoming evident that merely cutting out cigarettes, substituting unsaturated fats, and losing a few pounds may not achieve the desired effect unless these sacrifices are accompanied by a regular exercise program.

[244]

Physical activity not only burns off calories but also stimulates heart action, causing an increased blood supply to circulate through the system. Exercise helps to keep the arteries open, especially if they are already partly obstructed by excessive fat deposits. Just walking can help lower cholesterol levels and clear the arteries of plaques. For an example of what such a regimen can do for heart health, consider the Masai of central Africa.

To find a group of physically fit people practically free from heart disease has become an increasingly hard task in the civilized world. Yet one group that is remarkably blessed with this type of good health is the Masai tribe in Tanzania. A study supervised by George Mann, M.D., Sc.D., is published in *The Lancet* (December 25, 1955).

Great Walkers

Dr. Mann and his associates explain the habits of these people: "The environmental requirements of the Masai are rigorous. They spend much of their lives as boys walking with the herds. As warriors they are on the move almost daily, walking great distances in their surveillance of cattle, property, girls, and distant friends. Their exercise seems to be primarily walking which is done at a brisk, long stride" at a rate of three to five miles an hour.

The Masai are lean people. Despite a diet of meat and milk that is far from fat-free, they have low blood pressure, healthy arteries, and cholesterol levels lower than those of their vegetarian neighbors. The Masai

[245]

use no salt and in fact do not even have a word in the language for this dubious substance known to raise the blood pressure. Refined carbohydrates full of fat and sugar—cakes, cookies, candies—are completely unknown. Men do not smoke until age 30. Only a very small number of tribesmen have ever had jaundice, thyroid disorders, gout, or arthritis.

Dr. Mann examined the fitness of 53 Masai males between 14 and 64 years of age. The men were asked to walk on an electrically driven treadmill until they felt exhausted. After each man stopped, his pulse rate was counted. It was found that most of the subjects could outperform "athletes of Olympic standard." Even when the men did drop out, it was because of leg pain, rather than oxygen insufficiency. This experiment was a definite indication of a group in excellent physical shape with excellent heart conditions.

There is no reason why each of us cannot guard against death from a heart attack by changing certain habits. If you have a desk job or stay at home all the time, you are taking a risk. Dr. Mann cites the opinion of J. N. Norris: "Men in physically active jobs have less ischaemic heart disease during middle age, what disease they do have is less severe, and they develop it later than men in physically inactive jobs."

While regular exercise is the best preventive medicine for heart trouble, activity after a non-fatal attack is also beneficial. Dr. Joseph Wolffe, director of the Valley Forge Medical Center and Heart Hospital in Norristown, Pa., encourages recuperating patients to climb stairs. In a paper presented to the Annual Na-

[246]

tional Recreational Congress in Philadelphia, Pa., (1962), he wrote, "Stair walking involves all systems of the body. The body is carried upward by the skeletal muscles. Groups of muscles contract while their antagonists relax. The work that is required is not limited, however, to the lower extremities; important chemical changes take place, more blood and oxygen is needed by the active muscles. The heart and vessels are gradually strengthened to meet the demand."

Whether you are fit or unfit now, exercise can help prevent further deterioration of your arteries and can keep your circulatory system functioning well. Once you develop some kind of program, however, don't think that you can slip back into the alcohol, salt, sugar and nicotine habits. Exercise is most beneficial when the body is not overtaxed by these harmful substances which simply nullify the resistance you have tried to build up.

Will we ever be as healthy as the Masai? Such a dream may be possible if we change our ways. Although Dr. Mann admits that physical fitness has not been proved the only reason why the Masai do not succumb to heart disease, he concludes his study with this advice: "All of these facts indicate that coronary-heart disease, obesity, and diabetes, the prevalent chronic diseases of Western Society, are a consequence . . . of indolence and inactivity. . . . A great extension of data relating physical fitness to the prevention of these diseases is urgently needed."

[247]

CHAPTER XXX

Exercise -- What It Does

The most important thing that exercise does is to oxygenate the body, which is most desirable to a heart case, for it is lack of oxygen which is an important element in inducing a heart attack. Oxygenation of the body may be compared to the draft of a boiler which burns up the refuse and slag in the body.

Dr. Wm. B. Kountz, professor of clinical medicine at Washington University, at a public meeting recently said that the medical profession has long been aware that a decline in the body's oxygen consumption causes such ailments as hardening of the arteries, heart disease, body-wasting and other typical manifestations of old age. This is important, he said, in the maintaining of the burning or oxidative process of the body. *The Journal of the American Medical Association* of September 15, 1956, states that when the oxygen supply to the

[248]

tissues goes down, the number and size of the cells also decreases. This causes tissue atrophy, or aging. Thus, by taking exercise, and insuring the oxygenation of the body, one ages gracefully.

Another effect of oxygen was demonstrated by Dr. D. B. Hill of Harvard, who proved that the man who takes regular exercise requires "less oxygen to perform the same amount of work, mental or physical, than the man who does not" (*Time*, February 4, 1957). In other words, the person who takes daily exercise can turn out more work. Exercise also burns up sugar.

Angina pectoris, a disease marked by a sudden or periodic chest pain, sometimes with a feeling of suffocation and impending death, is due most often to lack of oxygen in the muscular substance of the heart; that is, the heart muscle.

Another effect of exercise is to maintain the general muscular tone throughout the body. This includes the heart muscle, the importance of whose tone can well be realized. An important muscle is the diaphragm which, if its muscular tone improves, will enable a person to breathe more efficiently. This means healthier lungs. The diaphragm is like the piston of a pump in its action, and if it has good tone, it can more efficiently cause the suction of blood into the heart via the great veins. Exercise breaks up congestion in the lungs. Breathing becomes easier.

The effect of exercise is to quicken the circulation. *Science News Letter* of November 3, 1951, says in this respect:

"In a man at rest about a gallon of blood is circulated every minute . . . approximately the entire blood supply visits the tissues once every minute. With vigorous exercise these visits may be eight or nine times as frequent. The blood, instead of traveling at a rate of 55 feet a minute in the large arteries may move 450 feet a minute. This makes possible a more rapid and complete removal of waste from all parts of the body, and increases the amount of oxygen in parts of the body depending on it. Exercise taken simply and regularly tends to keep the arteries soft, warding off arteriosclerosis or other old age conditions."

The aorta, one of the blood vessels that convey blood to and from the heart, will maintain a more even flow of blood if it becomes more elastic through exercise. It is through the compression of the veins that blood is pumped into the heart. Good muscular tone causes them to do this job better. Good muscular structure will also prevent a blood clot.

The veins have valves which are there to stop the blood from going the wrong way. If the muscular structure is good, the veins have good compression and are thus able to pump the blood to the heart more easily. If not, stasis, or a slackening of the blood flow, can occur.

Dr. Paul D. White, the President's heart specialist, in a medical article (*Journal of the American Medical Association,* Sept. 7, 1957) stated that exercise improves bowel function and digestion. It also helps to induce sleep, more "than any medicine, highball or television show." It controls obesity, and, most important, takes the fat out of the walls of the coronary

[250]

and other important arteries. This is one of the most important rewards of exercise. It reduces the cholesterol level of the blood.

Three doctors at the Sinai Hospital in Detroit proved this in experiments with rabbits. "The amount of atherosclerosis present in the exercise group at the end of that time appeared to be distinctly less than that in the sedentary group, and chemical tests (cholesterol) showed the same thing." This was written up in the *Proceedings of the Society for Experimental Biology and Medicine* (December, 1957). The same thing was shown in 20 men who were hard physical laborers and who also took a high caloric diet rich in fats. Their cholesterol level was lower than average (*Journal of the American Medical Association*, September 22, 1956, p. 423).

According to the *British Medical Journal* (October 22, 1955) the low cholesterol levels found in Guatemalans and Africans are not attributed to their limited diets but to the muscular activity and energy expenditure required in these cultures. "Reflection will show that such an explanation is at least as compatible with the available observations as is the dietary fat explanation which has been so widely advocated. When this effect of exercise was examined experimentally in human subjects, it was found that doubling the calorie intake of young men who were consuming a very high fat diet did not increase the serum cholesterol or lipoprotein levels so long as the excess energy was expended in physical activity."

Besides lowering the cholesterol level of the blood,

[251]

exercise increases the specific gravity of the body, making the tissues more compact. This is highly desirable in connection with the body's general economy, but especially in regard to the functioning of the heart. The subject was fully discussed in an earlier chapter of this series.

Dr. William Brady, in the *Chicago Daily News* of January 2, 1958, says that daily exercise—a brisk walk of several miles—causes the body to store up calcium. (See section on calcium and its importance to the action of the heart.) In other words, walking or other exercise promotes calcium metabolism. The reverse, says Dr. Brady, is also true. Prolonged confinement to bed or too much resting depletes the calcium reserve. That is why in so many cases a hip is broken after a bed-fast patient begins to move about. Many very old persons fall down and it is thought that as a result they break their hips. Now it is believed that the hip is broken first, which then causes the fall.

Exercise causes added vitamins to be absorbed by the body, especially vitamin A (*Journal of Nutrition*, April 10, 1958). This is probably due to better oxygenation and through improved digestion.

Exercise causes all the glands to secrete their hormones, digestive acids, enzymes and other substances. For example, after a few moments of walking, the adrenal cortex gland begins to secrete cortisone. Is it possible that lack of exercise, and the failure to secrete sufficient cortisone, is one of the causes of arthritis? Then artificial cortisone is given, but it is nothing like the original natural product produced by the adrenal

[252]

cortex, and in many cases causes dangerous side-effects. The substances secreted by the adrenal cortex feed the brain. Thus, walking or other exercise could well be a valuable stimulation to better mental activity.

According to the *Journal of the American Medical Association* (October 5, 1957), "The greatest value (of exercise) lies in its stimulating effect on endocrine (glands) activity, perhaps the thyroid in particular, and in overcoming the tendency to sleep and snooze, too much a counterpart of obesity." When the endocrine glands are reduced in efficiency, a common occurrence with old people, it contributes to the fatigue of old age, which shows the importance of regular exercise for older persons.

Soviet doctor Vladimir Filatov in *My Path in Science,* in speaking about glaucoma, where the main symptom is increased tension inside the eyeball, said, "Another useful auxiliary treatment is increased muscular activity. I pointed out the value of this method for the regulation of intra-ocular tension as early as 1937. Observations on a number of patients showed lowering of the intra-ocular tension after long walks."

Dr. Paul Dudley White, the President's heart physician, in the *New York Times Magazine,* June 23, 1957, said: "Another part of the circulatory apparatus helped by exercise is that of the smallest blood vessels, arterioles, capillaries and venules, which are rendered more active in their function by their response to regular exercise. The peripheral vessels of the hands, the feet and the ears react beneficially with less likelihood of sluggishness and stasis (a stopping of the circulation)."

[253]

There isn't a part of the body that doesn't seem to be aided by exercise and muscular activity.

Dr. William T. Foley of the New York Hospital, Cornell Medical Center, has worked out a "walking cure" for gangrene of the feet and legs. Says the *Science News Letter* of June 1, 1957, "Amputations were avoided and the gangrenous condition healed in 21 out of 22 cases when the patients got out of bed and walked around in spite of the ailment. . . . The gangrene was a complication of various circulatory diseases that had cut down the flow of the blood to the feet or legs. The customary practice is to keep such patients in bed and off their feet, but then the blood flow decreases even further and muscles begin to shrivel up.

"Along with the rest of the medical profession," Dr. Foley says, "we were hesitant to allow patients with gangrenous limbs to walk. The success of our surgical colleagues, however, in the treatment of fractures by exercise suggested that we might profit by their experience." So—even fractures are helped by exercise. Dr. Foley prohibits smoking in gangrene, since it constricts blood vessels and may cause the gangrene to return.

Another very desirable effect of exercise is the reduction of the pulse if it is too high. (This subject is covered in the chapters on the pulse.) A high pulse is an invitation to a heart attack, and should not be tolerated by a heart case. With a little effort you can control your pulse.

An important consequence of exercise is the enlargement of the coronary arteries. *The Lancet*, December 12, 1953, p. 1261, says, "The more you exercise, the

[254]

bigger your coronary arteries; the more you exercise, the faster the blood flows through them and the more difficult it is for an obstruction to develop on the walls." This authority says further, "I have for some time been considering various exercises with a view to providing the optimum coronary protection. I think skipping is the best, but people are intolerant of it, and, for the ordinary person, dancing of the Scottish country type is the most practicable proposition."

Earl Ubell, science editor of the *New York Herald Tribune* (July 7, 1957), said, "It is possible that exercise can increase the number of branches of the coronary artery going into the heart and provide additional channels for blood flow in case one of the vessels becomes blocked with the fatty substances like cholesterol." Dr. C. F. Wilkinson of the New York University Post Graduate School of Medicine, in the Allentown, Pa., *Evening Chronicle* (February 19, 1958) stated, "The arteries which feed the heart do not connect with each other, so if one of these vessels is blocked quickly, the muscle which feeds it receives no blood. If, however, the blockage is slow, the heart changes its blood vessel pattern by forming connections between the narrow vessel and another one. These connections cannot be formed rapidly.

"If an individual has been taking a relatively constant amount of exercise over a period of years, and has had a slow narrowing of the coronary arteries, it is quite likely that he has formed these connecting vessels."

Dr. Richard W. Eckstein of Western Reserve Uni-

[255]

versity, Cleveland, Ohio, working with a group of animals, showed that "when the artery which winds around the top of the heart is narrowed in dogs, collateral growth is improved by exercise." *The Medical Journal of Australia* (May 17, 1958) states, "The capillary network of athletes' hearts is unusually richly developed." The article says also, "It has been said that man's first mistake was the wheel . . . while it would undoubtedly be better for the general health if everybody used their muscles—cardiac and skeletal— to a much greater extent than is usual in the wealthier countries, it is doubtful whether this will happen on any large scale, and modern medicine must develop some other means of compensating for the disturbed central nervous and peripheral neurovegetative equilibrium if we want to escape further degeneration. Meanwhile, common sense says: 'Exercise.'" In fact, the data in this chapter would certainly indicate that, if you are a heart case, the height of common sense would be to be sure to exercise every day.

CHAPTER XXXI

Sex and the Middle-Aged Heart

When a man reaches middle age and thereafter, he will almost certainly find himself wondering at one time or another, "Is it safe for me to enjoy sex the way I did when I was younger?" If he has suffered a heart attack, the question takes on enormous significance. After all, rumors have been around for some time that sex can be fatal.

The Roman scholar Pliny may have been the first to start the rumor that sex relations can bring about a heart attack. Attila the Hun is said to have died while making love. The French sixteenth century essayist Montaigne claimed that a number of political figures died while in the midst of the embrace.

More recently, the Japanese *Journal of Legal Medi-*

cine (September, 1963) reported on 5,559 cases of sudden death over a four and a half year period. Dr. Masahiko Ueno, a Japanese pathologist, wrote that 34 of these cases were related to sexual activity. The Japanese have coined a word for this sort of thing, which is literally interpreted, "Death on top of tummy."

Surprisingly, only five of the victims were in their sixties. Twenty-one were from their early twenties to late forties. Eight were in their fifties.

But what does this study prove? How does it fit in with other findings? Myron Brenton, in his recent book *Sex and Your Heart* (Coward-McCann, Inc., 1968) explains in one curt sentence why it is so difficult to answer those questions: "Thick tomes on heart disease devote a paragraph, a page at most, to sex and the heart." Brenton says this condition exists "despite the fact that sex is one of the most basic and oft-performed of all human activities, and despite the fact, too, that during intercourse and especially at orgasm the heart pounds, the pulse quickens, the breath comes fast."

Several cases of heart attacks during coitus were reported informally by George Trimble, M.D., in the June 7, 1965 *Journal of the American Medical Association*. (Before that, reports of such death were virtually nonexistent, even in the medical literature.) Trimble wrote, "An Illinois physician tells of an instance of 'coronary attack' during sexual intercourse which attack he related to a 'strenuous psychoanalytic session' nine hours previously. An assistant medical examiner in Philadelphia believes there is a significant incidence of myocardial infarction (heart attack) associated with

[258]

coitus, but he has found it difficult to elicit background information to support this thesis."

Trimble also cites a case described by a Texas physician: "On 18 November 1958, at about 1:00 a.m. a 56-year-old white male, with a past history of myocardial infarction and cerebral arteriosclerosis with hemiparesis, (muscular weakness in one side of the body) was engaging in coitus when he suddenly rolled over on his back and rapidly and quietly expired."

Before Trimble's report, Dr. H. Alexander Heggtveit of the University of Ottawa Faculty of Medicine reported in the March 14, 1964 *Journal of the American Medical Association* on a 23-year-old soldier "who died while in bed with a woman of questionable character." Autopsy showed the boy had a severe case of coronary atherosclerosis. A similar study was reported in the November, 1956, *Journal of Applied Physiology.*

But none of these studies shed light on the question: "Is sex bad for the heart?" What they do suggest, in fact, is that each of the victims suffered heart disease all along, and if the fatal moment hadn't occurred when it did, it would have occurred anyway under some other strenuous circumstances not long thereafter.

Highly Accelerated Heartbeat

One of the earliest efforts to find out precisely what effect sex has on the heart was made in 1928 by Drs. Ernest P. Boas and Ernest F. Goldschmidt. Their findings were published in *The Heart Rate* published in 1932 by Charles C. Thomas. The heart beats and

[259]

respiratory rates of a married couple engaging in sex relations were recorded.

The findings were astounding. At climax, the couple's heartbeats reached 148.5 beats per minute—2½ beats per second! The average heartbeat rate is about 70 per minute. The man's heartbeat remained above 125 beats a minute for more than 20 minutes.

Studies by William H. Masters, M.D., and Virginia Johnson of the Reproductive Biology Research Foundation in St. Louis, Missouri, published in 1966 (*Human Sexual Response,* Little, Brown & Co.) were the most detailed yet conducted on the body's responses to the stresses of sexual relations. The researchers found that breathing rates exceed 40 per minute. They found heartbeats that sometimes exceeded 180 per minute or 3 beats per second.

Blood pressure is also radically affected. Although normal systolic pressure levels are usually 110 to 140 mm. Hg., they reached as much as 80 points above those figures. Diastolic elevation went from the norm of 70-96 to above 120. Facts such as these certainly indicate that sexual activity is extremely strenuous and would seem to point to danger for anyone with a heart condition.

But, as a matter of fact, no one can at this time make a statement about the matter authoritatively. Dr. Masters, who is perhaps the world's greatest authority on the physiology of sex, said in his recent book, "Clinicians daily face the problem of advising the patient recovering from an acute episode of coronary artery occlusion. One of the immediate problems is

[260]

that of the family unit's interest in returning to an active sexual relationship. How much cardiac strain develops in response to sexual tensions? . . . Are there sex techniques that will place less strain on the heart, yet relieve the individual and the family of their tension increment? These are but a few of the questions that medicine must answer."

But, as yet, they are not answered. Right now Masters and Johnson are carrying on further studies which they expect will shed light on this whole area—but findings will not be available for several years.

Doctors Avoid the Issue

In the meantime, most doctors simply avoid the issue. Richard H. Klemer indicated in the November, 1966 *Postgraduate Medicine* that physicians often fail to discuss sexual problems with patients, and this is as true with heart disease victims as it is with any other. Said Klemer, "Inadequate sexual communication is frequently the result of the physicians' own hesitant uneasiness."

That fact was amply illustrated through research conducted at the Pittsburgh Cardiac Work Evaluation Unit some years ago by Dr. William D. Tuttle. In a study of 39 cases of heart disease, in 27, doctors avoided giving any advice whatsoever regarding sexual activity. And of the 12 who did discuss sex with their patients, all were vague and unspecific with their advice.

Even today, no one has the last word on whether or not sex is permissible for a victim of a heart attack. At every medical convention, doctors will gather, choose up sides and argue with their viewpoints vigorously. But some facts are available. More, in fact, than the average person—even the average physician—realizes. And although these facts do not offer all the answers, they do shed some important light on the question, and suggest meaningful answers.

Illicit Love More Dangerous

One of these facts is that the overwhelming majority of sex-related heart attacks occur during affairs with paramours or prostitutes. The heightened excitement of a relationship with a new partner, coupled with the apprehension involved in an illicit situation, apparently placed an unnatural burden upon the heart in these cases.

That was the cause of a recent death in a north-eastern Pennsylvania motel. A middle-aged business-man who had asked a desk man to supply him with female companionship for the evening was so shocked when his daughter walked into the room to answer his request that he promptly dropped dead.

Just *how* seriously emotions affect the heart is illustrated in an article by Sidney B. Weinberg and M. Helpern, "Circumstances Relating to Sudden Unexpected Death in Coronary Heart Disease." It appeared in the book *Work and the Heart* by F. F. Rosenbaum, *et al.* (New York: Paul B. Hober, Inc., 1959). In studying 428 deaths related to heart disease, they found that many victims had experienced emotional crises just prior to death. One victim was a delicatessen owner who had been robbed. Another was a salesman being questioned by police about a robbery. Another died upon hearing of the death of a friend.

This may very well have been the case in the majority of the 39 heart attack victims studied by Dr. Tuttle at the Pittsburgh Cardiac Work Evaluation Unit to which we referred before. Yet, although many of the men may have suffered considerable emotional stress through leading a life void of sexual expression, the sex lives of two-thirds of these men were radically reduced because they feared—and their doctors did not correct the fear—that sex could bring on another heart attack.

Not all people react the same to sexual relations— and in fact, the same person does not always react in the same way. The emotions involved radically affect body reactions, and these emotions can vary widely. Under certain circumstances, for example, when a man is making love to his wife of many years he may feel only mild excitement. Under other circumstances, he may be enthralled in passion.

The variation in emotion radically affects the rate at which blood clots or thins. It affects cholesterol level. It causes blood vessels to constrict or expand. In each of these cases, the degree of excitement dictates the amount of work the heart will have to do.

Celibacy Causes Emotional Stress

Obviously, under some circumstances, sex can be very strenuous to the heart. But there is another side to the coin. Since sex is a biological fact of life, and a necessary fact at that, lack of sexual expression can

[263]

also be a cause of emotional stress. It hardly makes sense to tell a man who is tense, irritable and frustrated because of a lack of sexual gratification that he dare not seek relief because it will be bad for his heart. The tension of frustration can very well be worse.

The truth seems to be that *strenuous* sex, not sex itself, does realistically threaten the man with a weak heart. But anyone with an imagination, a willing companion and a helpful physician can soon develop a sexual technique which will keep stress at a minimum.

Brenton, in his book, gives these pointers:

1. Hazards lie in extremes of temperature. The heart has to work a good deal harder to keep body temperature normal when surrounding temperatures are extremely hot or extremely cold. Heavy sexual activities in extremes of temperature could overburden the heart and lead to an attack.

2. Hazards lie in heavy eating. For many years college students have avoided eating meals before exams. The idea is based on the sound medical knowledge that the digestive process requires a great deal of blood— and so does thinking. If the blood is needed in the stomach, the major supplies will not be sent to the brain and the mind will not work at optimum efficiency.

That fact explains why heavy eating should be avoided before sexual relations. Coitus demands heavy blood supplies in the pelvic area, and the stress of sending blood to both stomach and pelvic area simultaneously may be too much for a weak heart.

3. Hazards lie in too much drinking. Alcohol is a

[264]

cardiac stimulant and therefore causes the heart to work harder. It also loosens inhibitions, and may lead the person with an already weak heart to engage excessively in sex relations.

4. There are hazards in fatigue. Some doctors recommend a nap before sex because it avoids exhaustion. Fatigue is an additional needless handicap to impose on a heart that is already not working correctly.

5. Additional hazards lie in tension and fear. For some people, having sex following a heart attack is fraught with all kinds of anxieties. For them, certainly the lesser evil is to avoid the problem by abstinence. For others, sex relations are a means of proving something—masculinity, youth, health, etc. To succeed in bed becomes the big thing. Again, it is fraught with emotional stress, tensions and anxieties.

These emotional hazards are far more dangerous than the sex act itself. It is of great importance that anyone recuperating from a heart attack avoid approaching sex in such a tortured frame of mind.

Warning Signs

What we are saying is that sex, like anything else in life, should be approached with moderation—especially by anyone recuperating from a heart attack. When it is approached in this way, there is no need to feel that sex is any more dangerous than a slow walk in the park. The smart man, however, will keep in mind a few warning signs:

Chest pains during or after sex could mean the heart has been overexerted.

[265]

If heart palpitations continue for more than 15 minutes after sexual relations have ended, it may be time to call the doctor.

Shortness of breath ought not to last for more than 15 minutes, either.

Sleeplessness following sexual activity and apparently directly related to it is a warning sign.

Exhaustion the day after sexual activity indicates poor circulation—a heart that is not functioning well.

Even these indications are not conclusive. They may be totally unimportant, but they do indicate that a check-up is needed.

If these signs are absent, there is no reason at all why anyone—whether or not he has suffered a heart attack —should not have a satisfactory sex life. The guideline is summarized in a wise old proverb: All things in moderation;—which is not the same, by any means, as total abstinence.

CHAPTER XXXII

Exercise For a Stronger Heart

Often when a man reaches middle age he begins refraining from sexual activity, not because he no longer desires it, but because he is afraid of the exertion involved. And there is some basis for that concern, for, as we have pointed out, when coitus is prolonged and strenuous, it is certainly a physically taxing activity.

"A strong, healthy heart and an efficiently working circulatory system are as important to the act of sexual intercourse as they are to an Olympic athlete running the 100 meter sprint, and (it is) every bit as taxing," says Edward O'Relly in *Sexercises* (Crown, 1968). "This was most dramatically shown by tests carried out at the National Institutes of Health to determine the physiological costs of the sex act. Married couples, tested by scientific instruments, showed an increase of heartbeats from as low as 70 per minute to as high as 192 per minute in less than sixty seconds, with a tripling in breathing rate. This is comparable to the most vigorous athletic endeavor."

If you are not sure that you have a healthy heart and efficiently working circulatory system and are dubious about sex relations for that reason, what you need is a special program to prepare you for an active life —both sexually and otherwise. Such a program does exist. It is not a secret imported from the Orient. It is not patented. It does not cost money. And the Russians, believe it or not, did not invent it.

It is known as exercise. Practiced routinely and effectively, it seems to be the most effective heart disease preventive yet discovered.

What's more, the President's Council on Physical Fitness recently reported that even sexual potency can be increased through exercise.

But exercise, for all its value, is sorely lacking in the lives of most Americans. O'Relly, a prominent physical educationist who has made a lengthy study of the subject, writes:

"Automation and mechanization are robbing us of our health, strength, stamina, flexibility, vigor, agility, and neuromuscular coordination. Never in the entire history of mankind has there been such a great need for physical fitness, and with the development of each new labor-saving device, this need becomes increasingly greater.

Inactivity Leads to Degeneration

"Machines are replacing human muscles. Planes,

[268]

trains, automobiles and escalators are making legs almost useless. We are rapidly degenerating into a race of button-pushers. Most of our waking hours are spent on our posteriors—sitting, driving, watching, riding and otherwise engaged in sedentary pursuits. What with TV and spectator sports, even our recreation is becoming predominantly passive."

A lack of exercise is not only a major factor in the development of heart disease—it also can lead to a waning and inadequate sex life. Many studies have shown conclusively that exercise keeps the body young, vigorous and well-toned. One study showed that dogs forced to run on a treadmill survived their lazy mates. Geriatrics researcher Dr. Edward L. Bortz said, "We take vigorous exception to the prophets of gloom who see only the degeneration of the human body with the passing of time. It begins to appear that exercise is the master conditioner for the healthy and the major therapy for the ill."

For those men who are avoiding sex because of fear that it will damage their hearts, such avoidance—along with avoiding all other forms of exercise—may actually be self-defeating. There is some evidence that coitus itself has considerable benefit as an exercise. And it is the lack of exercise rather than its indulgence which leads to heart disease.

Perhaps the most convincing of all heart disease-exercise research projects are the Framingham study and the HIP study of 110,000 people covered by the Health Insurance Plan of Greater New York. In Framingham the researchers followed the health of more

[269]

than 5,000 adult residents for more than 10 years and found that "the most sedentary had a distinctly worse outlook" than those who were moderately active. They suffered more heart attacks and the attacks were more likely to be fatal.

Based on the findings of the HIP study, the scientists reported that a first heart attack, whether or not it is related to sexual activity, is more prevalent in physically inactive men than in men who are more active. That is true among both cigarette smokers and non-smokers. Men suffering a first myocardial infarction in the course of the study were divided into walkers and non-walkers. Fifty-seven per cent of those who neither walked nor engaged in other forms of physical activity were dead within 4 weeks, as compared with only 16 per cent of those who both walked and exercised in other ways.

Heart Muscle Requires Use

The heart is primarily muscle, and like other muscles, requires use. It also needs oxygen. Exercise enables the lungs to operate more efficiently, thereby delivering more oxygen through the coronary arteries to the heart. That plentiful supply of oxygen enables the heart to function at a lower blood pressure without having to work as hard.

One of the more widely reported effects of physical activity on the functioning of the heart is the development of extra circulation routes when main coronary artery branches become blocked. According to Dr. William B. Kannel of Harvard University, cited in O'Relly's book, "Persons who have an important de-

[270]

gree of blockage of the coronary artery, but continue to be physically active, can reasonably be expected to develop more collateral circulation than those with comparable coronary involvement who remain inactive." Dr. Richard Eckstein of Western Reserve University showed recently that exercise enabled dogs to develop collateral circulation even though their arteries were narrowed through surgery. The control animals who led sedentary lives developed no new pathways.

If you're convinced that exercise is necessary to assure a healthy heart, capable of sustaining sexuality and other normally vigorous activities, don't hold back because you can't decide which activities are best and how much should be done. Those problems have been solved for you. In a new book, *Aerobics* (M. Evans & Co., Inc., 1968), Drs. Kenneth H. Cooper and Kevin Brown of the U.S. Air Force Medical Corps explain that the best kind of exercise for cardiovascular health is that which demands oxygen and forces your body to process and deliver it. Running, swimming, cycling, walking, stationary running, handball, basketball and squash fall into that category. When you do those exercises, changes take place. Dr. Cooper calls it the training effect. For example, the lungs are conditioned to process more air with less effort, the heart grows stronger and pumps more blood with each stroke, the number and size of the blood vessels is improved.

How much do you require of those oxygen-demanding exercises (aerobics) and for how long? Dr. Cooper explains that through four years of studies on 5,000 officers and airmen he has been able to scientifically

[271]

measure the amount of energy all popular exercises cost the body to perform. Translating those amounts into points, he has established that a basic minimum of 30 points each week is necessary to produce and maintain cardiovascular health. The exercise sessions must take place at least 4 times a week, or every other day. And you can't earn the 30 points in one day and then forget about physical activity for the next six.

Fitness Test

In *Aerobics,* Dr. Cooper lists complete conditioning programs for each aerobic exercise, including the number of points you can earn. But before you can start gaining points by following one of the conditioning programs, it would be a good idea to take the Air Force 12-minute fitness test to see just what kind of shape you're in now. Your score on the test will determine how much or how long you have to exercise to gain your 30 points.

Before taking the test, it might be good to get your doctor's permission, especially if you're over 30. The test itself is simple, and only requires that you run as far as possible within 12 minutes. Of course if your breath gets short, walk for a while until it comes back and then run some more.

Measure off a certain running area of up to 2 miles. You may want to get permission to use the track at your local high school or Y.M.C.A. and take your test there. But wherever you take the test, try to run the whole time at a pace you can maintain without excessive strain. After you have run for 12 minutes, check your distance on the chart which follows.

Now you're ready to start getting your 30 points to keep in active and productive health. Six different progressive conditioning courses are listed in *Aerobics*. Chances are, if you have had little exercise in recent years and are over 30, you'll fall into the "very poor" category I. A conditioning course for that category is reprinted from the book.

At first, exercise may seem like a waste of time. But within six weeks that attitude will change. A definite improvement will be obvious. You will not tire quickly. In the winter months, when activities such as snow shoveling becomes necessary, you will not approach them with dread that a heart attack is imminent.

And when it comes to the marital relationship, fear of the stress involved will not be a problem for you.

CATEGORY 1

Week	Distance (miles)	Walk/run	Time Goal (minutes)	Freq/ Wk	Points/ Wk
1	1.0	WALK	13:30	5	10
2	1.0	WALK	13:00	5	10
3	1.0	WALK	12:45	5	10
4	1.0	W/R	11:45	5	15
5	1.0	W/R	11:00	5	15
6	1.0	W/R	10:30	5	15
7	1.0	RUN	9:45	5	20
8	1.0	RUN	9:30	5	20

9	1.0	RUN	9:15	5	20
10	1.0	RUN	9:00	3	
	and				21
	1.5	RUN	16:00	2	
11	1.0	RUN	8:45	3	
	and				21
	1.5	RUN	15:00	2	
12	1.0	RUN	8:30	3	
	and				24
	1.5	RUN	14:00	2	
13	1.0	RUN	8:15	3	
	and				24
	1.5	RUN	13:30	2	
14	1.0	RUN	7:55	3	
	and				27
	1.5	RUN	13:00	2	
15	1.0	RUN	7:45	2	
	and				
	1.5	RUN	12:30	2	30
	and				
	2.0	RUN	18:00	1	
16	1.5	RUN	11:55	2	
	and				31
	2.0	RUN	17:00	2	

Charts reprinted from *Aerobics* (M. Evans & Co., Inc.)

[274]

Part Seven:

THE PULSE

CHAPTER XXXIII

High Pulse Rate Is Dangerous

J. I. Rodale

In the consideration of heart disease one of the most important factors is the pulse (a high pulse being very dangerous in such a condition). Very little, however, is heard about this subject when heart disease is being discussed. In my treatment of the subject of heart disease I therefore intend to go into the subject of the pulse in some detail.

According to the *Encyclopedia Britannica,* "The normal average pulse rate is 72 per minute, in women about 80; but individual variations from 40-100 have been observed consistent with health. In the newborn the pulse beats on the average 130-140 times a minute; in a one-year-old child 120-130; three years 100; ten years 90; fifteen years 70-75. Active muscular exercise may increase the pulse rate to 130. Nervous excitement,

[277]

extreme debility and rise of body temperature also increase it markedly. The pulse is more frequent when one stands than when one sits, or lies down, and this is especially so in states of debility. The taking of food, increases it." In aging there is a very slow and gradual increase of the pulse so that in a person over 80 it might reach 80 beats a minute, or more.

When we use the word *pulse* we are talking about what is called the heart rate, or the rate at which the heart pumps the blood. While the body is at rest the heart will pump at an average rate of 90 gallons of blood an hour. During violent exercise it will pump at the rate of 450 to 600 gallons an hour, which means that the pulse goes up. But the rate at which the heart will pump differs in different people. For example, taking arbitrary figures, in one person it might take 100 beats to pump a gallon of blood while in another it might have to be done with 200 beats. The pulse beat represents the rate at which the heart pushes the blood through a network of vessels in the body that average 168 million miles in length. There are many factors involved in this work, which will be discussed, but I will state as a general rule that the lower the pulse, within reason of course, the better it is for the health of your heart.

Drs. Raymond Pearl and W. Eden Moffet, in a report to the National Academy of Sciences in 1940, reported that in studying the lives of 386 men, they found that those lived longer who had a lower pulse by about four beats a minute than the shorter-lived ones. The long-lived group lived on an average 26 years

[278]

longer than the short-lived group. Incidentally, the long-lived group had a weight of 6 pounds each less than the short-lived groups. The interesting fact in this study is that if only a 4 beat difference had such a significant effect, what would be the effect of a greater difference? For example, by certain methods, I reduced my own pulse from 85 to about 68. The method will be explained later.

The insurance companies are aware that people with high pulse rates will not live as long as those with average pulse rates and will accept few persons for insurance whose pulse rate is higher than 100.

According to the August 7, 1954 issue of the *Journal of the American Medical Association* (page 1328) a study conducted by the Society of Actuaries showed that in people with very high pulse rates, the number of deaths from cancer was about 60 per cent higher than the average, and the number of lung cancer deaths 150 per cent higher. The item stated, "There were similar findings among persons with significant heart murmurs." When we checked this item to the source we found that a high pulse rate in this study was 90 to 100.

Dr. E. P. Luongo of Los Angeles made a study of 100 coronary disease cases as compared to 200 people in good general health and made a startling discovery. Quoting the *Journal of the American Medical Association* (November 19, 1956), "Over two-thirds of the patients with coronary disease showed a sustained rise in pulse rate (15 to 30 beats per minute) and diastolic pressure (10 to 30 mm. Hg) on the average of two

[279]

to five years prior to attack. By contrast, only one-third of the control patients showed significant changes in pulse rate or diastolic pressure two to five years prior to this study."

In other words, if all people of middle age and over would keep a check of their pulse, let us say, taken weekly or monthly, many of them would note this warning, this increase of their pulse, given far in advance, and could take the necessary measures to bring it down and thus save their life. Dr. Luongo states that this elevation of the pulse is associated with nutrition, stress and sedentary habits, and advises that such rise in pulse should be treated in these categories, regardless of what the electrocardiogram shows. I like one statement that this author makes. He says, "Physicians, in the future, will need more scientific and systematized information on positive health measures as they relate to normal nutrition and the tailoring of individual exercise patterns." This doctor is ahead of his time.

Now suppose you suddenly discover that your pulse is high. Is there anything you can do about it? The answer is a definite yes. How does one go about reducing one's pulse? There are several things you can do.

First, you must reduce the quantity of food you eat per day. This should apply mainly to overweight persons so that if you are underweight, you would have to get special advice in this category. But ordinarily to eat less is just plain common sense. I would like to refer to an experiment that was done with water fleas, described in a book entitled *The Status of Food Enzymes in Digestion and Metabolism,* by Edward

[280]

Howell. When the diet of the fleas was limited as to quantity, their pulse or heart beat went down, and they lived longer. Of course, we are not water fleas; but there is much medical evidence that by lowering the quantity of food eaten, life can be prolonged. However, very little stress has been placed on the fact that this reduced the pulse.

A physician writes to the editor of a medical journal about a patient who is suffering from a high pulse. The editor advises, among other things, that the amount of food at the evening meal be reduced and cautions him to divide the total daily food intake into four or five small meals. There also is evidence that in serious cases of high pulse (tachycardia) fasting is effective in slowing down the heart action.

A second means of lowering the pulse is to avoid emotional storms. A 12th-century Persian essayist, Nizami Aruzi, describes Avicenna's knowledge of the effect of the emotions on the pulse, as follows:

"A young man related to Qabus, the ruler of Mazandaran, had fallen ill. The leading doctors of the town could not be of any help. Young Avicenna was called in, and after the usual medical tests he decided that the malady was not a physical one. However, the melancholic patient would not utter a word. Avicenna decided it was love-sickness and set out to discover the object of his love. He called in a man who knew the town well and asked him to repeat names of districts of the town while he held the patient's pulse. He discovered that when a certain district was mentioned, there was an increase in the pulse-rate. He then elimi-

[281]

nated all streets but one in that district and all houses but one in that street, using the same method. Thus he concluded that his patient was in love with a maiden at that particular house."

Of course, the small, petty irritations that are strewn in our daily paths do not mean much. What we must avoid are the more tumultuous storms. By this I mean such things as your wife's running away with another man, or your own losing a business through bankruptcy, or losing your entire fortune in a stockmarket crash— events that make some persons want to jump out of windows. These happenings cause the pulse rate really to go way up.

Dr. William Dock, professor of medicine at State University of New York College of Medicine, at a meeting of the New York Academy of Medicine in 1951 said, "Cardiac acceleration is a common sequel of anger, apprehension and related moods, so that heart failure may be precipitated by emotional storms, just as it is by fever and other conditions . . . which accelerate the pulse."

Therefore, if you do not wish to have emotional storms that will raise your pulse, so live that your wife will not want to run away with another, be careful and conservative in business, do not buy stocks on margin—own them outright and avoid purchasing stocks that are too speculative.

A third means of lowering the pulse, if one is a smoker, is to eliminate that habit. Nicotine causes a shrinking of the arteries and will raise the pulse from 5 to 20 beats a minute. There is so much evidence of this in medical literature that I will not devote more space to this aspect of the subject. But any smoker can prove it for himself. Just stop smoking for a day, taking the pulse before and after this period.

High temperature may raise the pulse. If a person has a heart condition he should not work in front of a steel furnace, or in a bakery where the heat is high. It will raise the pulse by 10 or more beats a minute. In a scientifically devised experiment a man went into a laboratory where the temperature was 104° F. At the end of an hour his pulse was beating 40 per cent faster than usual. After 2 hours it was up 70 per cent. That may be the reason why so many elderly persons die during a heat wave. Lives can be saved in such cases by air conditioning, or some other means of combatting the heat.

A test was made of a group of persons in Ceylon, which is a tropical country, and it was found that their average pulse rate was greater than that of people who inhabit more temperate climates. (*Ceylon Journal of Medical Science*, June, 1949.)

Fifth: Avoid the use of drugs. Physicians have observed very high pulses in persons taking antihistamines. Many persons take this type of drug for hay fever. Many sulfur-containing drugs will heighten the pulse. Digitalis, given to prevent a heart attack, has been known to accelerate the pulse. Desiccated thyroid substance will increase the heart rate, as will certain preparations used to cure the tobacco habit. A person can easily check the pulse effect of any drug he is tak-

[283]

ing. Most of them are bad for the pulse, which means bad for the heart.

Sixth: Sex relations will raise the pulse and bring it up to 150 or even more. In older persons with a weak heart they might make it jump much higher.

Calcium also has an effect on the pulse. Dr. Edward Podolsky, in the *Illinois Medical Journal* (August, 1939) cited a series of five cases in which through the administration of calcium a high pulse was "controlled with dramatic effectiveness, both to the patient's delight and the doctor's surprise." We suggest the use of bone meal tablets as the most natural and effective form of calcium available.

There are two other means of reducing the pulse which are extremely important. One is exercise, and the other is a study of one's diet to eliminate particular foods that have a propensity to raise the pulse. It is a form of allergy. The science of ascertaining these pulse-irritating foods was developed by Arthur F. Coca, M.D., and will be discussed in the following chapter along with a description of how I reduced my pulse by means of exercise. In connection with exercise, however, you must know that sudden exercise will raise the pulse, but if you take it every day, consistently, the jump in the pulse because of it will be less, and eventually it will reduce the resting pulse materially. A walk of an hour a day will accomplish wonders in reducing a high pulse.

In view of all these safe means of reducing a high pulse it is surprising to note that the medical profession still depends on drugs to do the job. Take a typical

[284]

case described in the *New York State Journal of Medicine*. A 65-year-old physician has had repeated attacks of tachycardia (high pulse), which often came after a period of excessive eating. "His family physician was able to control the attacks with sufficient morphine to produce narcosis (unconsciousness). Despite the usual routine the last attack persisted. He was given .8 mg. Lanatoside C. This dosage was repeated in one hour. Immediately after the second injection, the attack subsided abruptly. He had no toxic effects from the drug."

Three other cases are presented in which drugs are used effectively, but the trouble is, it is only palliation. The causes are not found and removed. The condition will recur. And it is easy to say that no toxic effects were observed. Such effects can take years to show themselves.

It is too bad that physicians do not concern themselves with more natural approaches to the attack of a disease. In that way they would learn more about the causes of such diseases.

Take the case of the famous surgeon who died of a heart attack upon shoveling snow after a hearty meal. He probably did not know much about the theory and action of the human pulse. He probably had a high pulse to begin with, no doubt due to smoking and leading a sedentary life. A heavy meal can add ten to fifteen beats per minute to the pulse. On top of that the exercise of shoveling snow added still more to it. If he happened to be suffering from a cold his pulse would be still higher, and more so if he was taking drugs for it. So the famous surgeon, who knows

[285]

how to perform beautiful operations, but who doesn't know the simplest facts about his own pulse, was killed by his own ignorance.

There are some cases that require medical attention. Sometimes a high pulse is associated with rheumatoid arthritis, or with hyperthyroidism (overactive thyroid). In such cases it is best to seek good medical attention. This is one of these emergency situations where even the most naturally-minded persons had better seek out a good doctor.

But it is remarkable what a person can accomplish himself in the case of a high pulse.

CHAPTER XXXIV

The Coca Method

J. I. Rodale

The method by which I reduced my pulse from 85 to 68 actually is a combination of two methods. One is a reduction in the pulse due to a campaign of consistent daily exercise. The other is by the Dr. Coca method of ascertaining particular foods that accelerate the pulse and eliminating them from one's diet.

Several years ago I was extremely fortunate in discovering Dr. Arthur F. Coca's work in curing allergies through the observation and control of the human pulse. Up to this time the procedure, in checking for a person's allergies, was to scratch the skin with a needle, but Dr. Coca obtained the same results, even more correctly, by observing the effect of each food on a person's pulse. If, when a person ate only of one

[287]

particular food, it was observed that it abnormally raised the pulse, then there was an allergy to that food. Dr. Coca found that the average sick person's pulse was high because in his diet there were usually included 5 or 6 foods which were difficult for his digestive system to handle, the theory being that in such cases the heart had to work harder to bring extra pressure to bear to complete the digestion of those foods.

In following Dr. Coca's system you choose a time about an hour and a half after you have eaten and eat a small portion of a food that you wish to test, taking your pulse immediately before the test. You then take your pulse a half hour later, and again a half hour after that, recording the figures in a ruled blank book, with the date, time, etc., leaving room for a list of the food eaten, and other comments. It will become a valuable record for later study. If the figures are kept on pieces of paper it is easy for them to get lost.

It is best to take your pulse-reading at the wrist, using two fingers. For variation I began to take my pulse recordings next to my ear, but after a few days, a peculiar feeling developed in that region, and I went back to the wrist.

I found that the average food raised the pulse from three to five points per minute, although there were some that did not raise it at all, but that when a food caused the pulse to run up 8 or 9 points, it was usually one of the allergy-causing ones. In my own case I discovered that figs, honeydew melon, hot chicken soup, onions, whole wheat and fried foods of any kinds were the basic trouble-makers. It was absolutely fascinating

[288]

the fun there was in checking them down. For example, at first the indication showed that chicken raised my pulse unduly. But after I had accumulated sufficient records, showing in each case whether the chicken had been fried or broiled, I found that my pulse went up only when I ate fried chicken. I could eat broiled chicken without any trouble at all.

In the case of wheat, I made a rather thorough study. I found that whole wheat bread raised my pulse, but white bread did not. I could also eat wheat germ, which is present in whole wheat and not in white bread, without having the pulse go up. I therefore concluded that it was the bran that was difficult for my stomach to handle. This would indicate that, for me, the best kind of bread would be one with everything in it but the bran—a branless whole wheat bread. I found, however, that I could tolerate raw wheat seed, even though it contained bran. I was allergic, therefore, only to cooked bran.

French fried potatoes would send my pulse up, but not mashed or baked potatoes with the skins. It was the oil used in frying that I seemed to have a difficulty in handling. I could eat cantaloupe but not honeydew, and regarding figs, I used to eat them by the pound. No wonder my pulse had been around 85 and sometimes 95.

I found that coffee did not raise my pulse even a point and was surprised. I am not a drinker of any alcoholic beverages but, just to test, I drank some Scotch and soda, and beer, and was amazed to find that such drinks also kept my pulse down.

[289]

Regarding coffee, I discovered that the way we made it, in glass, did not raise my pulse, but if boiled in an aluminum utensil, it *did* raise it unduly. In this respect I would like to mention that Dr. Coca had six patients whose pulses were raised by eating foods cooked in aluminum pots. He found also that stainless steel ware offended in some cases. Only enamel or glassware resulted in keeping the pulse down. Coca says further: "Vaughan in his *Practice of Allergy,* p. 831, mentions 'the cure of cases of long-standing refractory colitis following change from aluminum cooking utensils to enamel or glass vessels.'"

I checked the effect of meat on my pulse. In no case was it unfavorable. It is a known medical fact, incidentally, that meat does not have to be chewed much. It is the carbohydrates that need lots of work in the mouth. Bear in mind, however, that these idiosyncrasies with regard to food vary with different persons. I may have an allergy to figs, for example, while you might eat them with impunity, so it is important that you check yourself.

The whole thing is terrific in its implications! When one considers what a reduction of the pulse means to one's well-being and longevity, it is to wonder that so little work has been done in connection with researches on the human pulse. In my own case, merely by cutting certain items of food out of my diet, my pulse was reduced by 15 beats per minute. This means that every hour my pulse beat 60 x 15 or 900 times less. And in a full 24-hour day my heart had to expand and contract 900 x 24 less times or 21,600 less times a day.

[290]

Merely by eliminating a few foods that I can easily get along without, my heart saves 43,200 movements in only one day. This is 21,600 expansions and 21,600 contractions. The heart actually moves between one and two inches each time in such expansion and contraction. Can you visualize this? Try to open and close your fist 21,600 times, moving it each time from one to two inches.

This means a saving of 15,768,000 movements a year for my little old heart. Is it any wonder that Dr. Raymond Pearl found that people who die young on the average have high pulses?

It certainly will pay everyone who reads this to check his or her pulse, and if it is above 75 to try to discover what is raising it. In Coca's work he is able to bring patients' pulses down to as low as 65.

If you decide to make a pulse study, my suggestion is first, for about a week, to keep a record of your pulse before and after whole meals. Take the pulse a half hour and an hour after your regular meals, without attempting to cut anything out of your diet. Later, after you have learned what foods are irritating your pulse, and have eliminated them, do the same, and observe the difference in the pulse increase, before and after meals.

The Coca system is now available in a book called *The Pulse Test* by Arthur F. Coca, M.D., published by Lyle Stuart, New York, N.Y. In it Dr. Coca describes symptoms which sensationally disappeared when the pulse was lowered, in migraine, fatigue, nervousness, indigestion, dizziness, constipation, neu-

[291]

ralgia, canker sores, chronic rhinitis, heartburn, urti-
caria, epileptic seizures, overweight, psychic depression,
asthma, and many others. Dr. Coca has hundreds of
cured patients who will be eternally grateful to him
for restoring them to health by his pulse-reduction
method. Most of them were stubborn cases that had
resisted the usual medical treatments. Dr. Coca has
also written up his method in medical textbook form
for physicians. It was published by Charles C. Thomas
Co., medical textbook publishers, of Springfield, Illinois,
and is an extremely technical piece of work.

For a heart case it is of the utmost importance to
make use of the Coca system for reducing the pulse, for
the heart will have far less work to do if the pulse is
significantly lowered.

I would like to describe another bit of personal
research that was an outcome of my pulse experiments.
I noticed that after one particular meal my pulse shot
up much more than it should have, and for no account-
able reason. After a bit of reflection, however, I re-
called that I had overlooked taking my vitamins at
that meal. In other words, I figured, in some way,
vitamins added to food at meals cause it to be more
thoroughly digested.

What is the reasoning behind this statement? Digestion requires the aid of the pump—the heart. If there
is some difficulty at a particular meal, the heart has to
pump more, which is reflected in more beats of the
pump per minute. Could it be possible that vitamins
act as catalysts with food, causing it to be more
thoroughly digested and absorbed by the blood stream,

[292]

thus putting less of a load on the heart? If this is so, think what a help the taking of vitamins at meals could be to the average heart case! The important point at issue is, that if the results I have obtained are generally applicable, then it is extremely important that we divide our daily vitamin ration into three portions, taking some at breakfast, some at lunch, and some at dinner.

But, of course, one swallow does not make a summer, so I decided on a scientific experiment, more or less. I was going to eat a uniform lunch for ten successive days, but take vitamins only every other day. Before I ate my lunch I took my pulse and I took it again one-half hour after the end of the meal and again one hour after the end of the meal. I tried to have meals that were as uniform as possible, using meat-balls as the base of six lunches and broiled chicken for the other four. There were, of course, such things as peas, carrots, lettuce, fruit, parsley, etc.

In connection with the meat-balls I experienced some trouble. On my original check-up I had discovered that when I ate anything with onions my pulse would jump up unusually, and I found that the meat-balls, being made with onions, accounted for the big rise in the pulse in some of the meals with meat-balls. But since the onions were present in the meat *with* as well as *without* vitamins, the conditions were averaged out and did not distort the end results.

At the end of this chapter are appended in table form the details of the experiment. On the average, where vitamins were taken with the meals, one-half

[293]

hour afterward, my pulse had risen an average of only 3 3/5 beats per minute, whereas where vitamins were not taken it jumped by 7 2/5 beats or 105 per cent more. At one hour after the meals, where vitamins were taken the pulse rose by but 5 2/5 beats, but where they were not taken, the average jump at this time was 12 1/5 beats, or 126 per cent higher. These are extremely significant increases and in my own case show two things: one—it pays to take the vitamins I am taking. And two—it proves that I should take my vitamins with my meals.

I am sure that anyone will admit that the proper digestion of food is of extreme importance to the human body, because it is the first step in the chemical process which is at the bottom of all body processes. The raw materials for these processes must be in the proper condition, just as the building blocks must be, if a good building is to be erected. But I would like to draw attention to a certain condition in which it is extremely important that attention be given to perfect digestion of food, and that is obesity. In my opinion overweight, with few exceptions, can be usually attributed to two basic errors, overeating and defective digestion. The food is not thoroughly digested. Some people have referred in an amateur way to the fact that the food "does not get burned up," but they are on the right track, of course. The glands enter into the picture too.

All I know is that as soon as I began to take fairly good doses of natural vitamins and reduced my intake of food somewhat, such a startling change occurred in

[294]

my appearance, due to the reduced weight, that I must attribute the greater part of it to the vitamins and to the better digestion of my food, due to the fact that I took my vitamins at mealtime. And I must say that it was pleasant music to hear the ah's and the oh's of my friends, some of whom accused me of taking reducing pills.

What I wish to imply here is that it may be generally possible, if people will reduce, to take a whole array of natural vitamins at meals, that, due to the better digestion, or due to some hidden factor produced by the vitamins, there may be an improvement in the biological set-up which will prevent that haggard, face-drawn appearance so common in reducers. At least that is what happened to me, and I offer it for all it is worth. I might also say that I can now eat more than I used to without it all immediately turning into fat. You mustn't forget, of course, that I usually walk an hour a day. Perhaps that is part of the biologic process.

There may be some who will say that the whole experiment was unbalanced by the fact that I knew what I was doing, that my mind, therefore, affected the pulse by the power of mind over matter. But they should bear in mind that when I originally noted the big jump in my pulse, before this experiment was attempted, it was only later that I discovered it was due to not having taken my vitamins at that meal.

Here are the mathematical results of my experiment. (see chart)

I did a few experiments, altering the combination of vitamins and checking each vitamin separately. Some

[295]

worked, while others did not. But bone meal was effective every time in keeping the pulse from rising too much. This is in keeping with researches already referred to, indicating that calcium is effective in lowering the pulse. Taking bone meal, therefore, is a must to everyone who wishes to keep his pulse within decent bounds.

And to keep the pulse within bounds may be a life and death matter. In this connection, I am reminded of the story about a famous Boston surgeon who was making the rounds at the hospital. Suddenly an old man called him to his bedside and asked, "Tell me, Doctor, how do I feel?"

The doctor carefully took the old man's pulse. Then he said, "I have good news for you. You're feeling fine."

The old man smiled with relief. "Thank God," he said.

Vitamin vs. No Vitamin Pulse Readings

	Meals With No Vitamins			Meals With Vitamins		
Date—1956	Pulse at Start	½ Hour After Meal	1 Hour After Meal	Pulse at Start	½ Hour After Meal	1 Hour After Meal
Feb. 14	72	82	90	..	..	..
15	..	..	..	76	84	84
16	76	90	84	..	..	..
17	..	..	..	73	76	85
18	72	72	77	..	..	..
19	..	..	..	68	72	70
20	70	75	90	..	..	..
21	..	..	..	73	74	74
22	68	76	78	..	..	..
23	..	..	..	72	74	76
Total	358	395	419	363	380	389
Average	71 3/5	79	83 4/5	72 2/5	76	77 4/5

[296]

With Vitamins
  ½ hr. (72 2/5 from 76 = 3 3/5)
Without Vitamins
  ½ hr. (71 3/5 from 79 = 7 2/5)
  _____
Net Increase   3 4/5
                      _____
                      105%

With Vitamins
  1 hr. (72 2/5 from 77 4/5 = 5 2/5)
Without Vitamins
  1 hr. (71 3/5 from 83 4/4 = 12 1/5)
  _____
Net Increase   6 4/5
                      _____
                      126%

[297]

CHAPTER XXXV

The Reduction of Pulse by Exercise

J. I. Rodale

The second method by which I brought my pulse rate down was by exercise.

Before I became aware of the power of exercise to bring the pulse down I was the most typical example of the sedentary businessman you could find. But after writing my series called *This Pace Is Not Killing Us,* I began to realize that unless I went in for exercise, my physically inactive life would surely kill *me* before my time.

But here I was with a high pulse which had to come down by means of exercise, or else my life would be shortened, and, on the other hand, a heart condition which might not respond too well to exercise. I had always heard that a heart case must rest as much as possible. So I decided to approach the matter warily. The first day I walked for only 10 minutes. Nothing happened! I was still alive. For the next few days I walked 10 minutes each day. Then I upped it to 15 and in about a week I was doing a full hour every morning, covering a brisk 3 miles, and enjoying it immensely.

One day during this hourly walk it seemed that my heart began to pound a little, so I stopped and took my pulse. To my surprise I found it to be 112. As my pulse at rest was between 76 and 80, I came to the conclusion that it was the exercise of walking that was making my heart work harder. A few hours later at rest my pulse was back to about 78. In other words, the demands that my walking made on my heart had raised it about 35 beats a minute. An interesting bit of knowledge, I thought.

Thinking that danger might be concealed somewhere in this fact, I decided from this point on to keep a record of my pulse during these walks. I did it scientifically, that is, I took it eleven times during the hour, at exact predetermined spots, so that the comparative daily record would mean something. Each day I added up the eleven figures and divided by eleven. Here are the average daily pulse results for the seven weeks of record keeping:

July 12	95.6		15	98.5
13	101.0		16	94.1
14	97.5		17	94.8

[299]

18	96.1	12	97.5
19	96.7	13	——
20	97.7	14	86.6
21	96.1	15	86.0
22	96.3	16	86.3
23	93.3	17	84.8
24	93.6	18	91.4
25	94.4	19	90.7
26	——	20	96.7
27	93.8	21	90.0
28	94.4	22	85.4
29	87.0	23	83.6
30	89.8	24	85.1
31	92.3	25	84.5
August 7	90.9	26	83.4
8	87.4	27	84.7
9	——	28	82.7
10	87.3	29	81.3
11	86.7	30	80.7

For those who do not like to analyze figures, I have made a chart. Note the remarkable reduction in the last few readings. To me this is nothing short of miraculous. After only seven weeks, I could walk an hour with my pulse about 13 beats per minute less than its high at the beginning of this period. I can also say that after the second week I began to finish off the walk with a wonderful feeling of euphoria, with no pounding of the heart. I would feel thoroughly relaxed with no suffering of fatigue or exhaustion.

A word about the method of taking my pulse. When

I stop, I wait about twenty seconds, and then count the beats of my heart as I note the ticking off of 30 seconds by the watch. I then take the count of the next 30 seconds and that is the one I record. This, of course, is then multiplied by two. I stop for a rest of about a half minute to a minute, halfway between each pulse stop, thus making about 20 stops in all. However, if I experience any pressure symptoms I will stop for a moment wherever necessary. Remember, I am still a heart case.

The most unusual thing of all is that in the last six days my chest pressure symptoms all but disappeared. For the first five weeks or so I continued to experience these symptoms—more on some days, and less on others, but I felt them only in the first 15 minutes of walking, as this part of the walk contains several up-grades. After this first quarter of an hour I could make the other hills with rarely a pressure pain. Evidently by this time the body has become thoroughly oxygenated, and the physical exercise has caused the blood to flow more vigorously through the coronary arteries.

But, in the last six days there were practically no pressure symptoms even during the first 15 minutes, and you can imagine how I felt about it. It will be sensational if this keeps up. If I never again experience the pressure pains on movement of any kind, it would be stupendous! And, of course, it would add to my life. Is it possible that I will be absolutely cured? I cannot believe it, but will continue with this experiment. As long as I am physically able, and the elements permit, I will walk my brisk hour and more every day.

[301]

It is interesting to study the chart and to note the successive waves, each one going lower than its predecessor. With regard to the sudden leap upwards of August 18, 19, 20, I have a theory. In order to explain it, may I say that during all these walks I found no direct relationship between the experiencing of a chest pressure symptom and the pulse at that moment. I could have a low pulse when there was a chest pain, and a high pulse when there was none, or vice versa. Now, it was beginning with the morning of August 17, the start of the period of the banishment of heart pressure symptoms, that my pulse suddenly began to shoot upwards. For three days it kept leaping. This set me to wondering. What could be the reason for it? I have come up with a possible explanation, although I know that it is rank theory. But it is worthwhile talking about it.

As my walks progressed, from day to day, there occurred a reduction in the pulse, and a development gradually of a sense of well-being towards the end of each walk. This indicated possibly that the flabbiness of the heart was turning into muscle. But there was still something wrong either with the heart, or the arteries leading in and out of it, that gave me the pains during the first fifteen minutes of walking each day. Then these practically disappeared, and at the same time there is a sizeable increase in the pulse. Does this indicate a second step in the rebuilding process? Have they been able to close some kind of gap? Have they engaged in some additional physical building of something in the heart, an action which required the help

[302]

of the whole heart to pump more blood for its accomplishment? Such a project would definitely raise the pulse.

Then the thing is done. The heart goes back to its previous pace. It goes down as precipitately as it went up. Is this fantastic reasoning? Perhaps. But it will have to do until someone works out a better reason. Perhaps it was not the heart alone. Is it possible that my lungs were strengthening themselves, being able to perform more efficiently so as to give more oxygen to the heart with less physical action of taking breaths? Is it possible that on August 17 something physical happened with regard to my lungs, something that knitted together something in which the heart had to take part by furnishing more blood for the building?

It is interesting to be aware that when a man-made machine has to be fixed, it must stop working, and outside forces do the job. But the heart performs the job of reconstruction itself and at the same time it must continue to pump blood to the rest of the organs of the body.

One more observation. Toward the end of the test I noticed that the pulse during the second half minute of its taking went down more than it used to. Before this, the pulse in the second period would be almost as high as that of the first. It indicates a newly acquired ability of the heart to snap back to normal after exertion. I note also that I breathe better while working at my desk.

During my daily walk, I perspire profusely. Perspiration is one means the body employs to rid itself of tox-

[303]

ins, or poisons. Is it possible that such poisons, remaining in the body, because of a sedentary daily regimen, make the heart work harder to rid the body of them through other means and channels?

Is it also possible that these toxins by remaining in the body and distorting the blood chemistry on a permanent, continuing basis, further interfere with various internal processes, which throw additional strain onto the heart, thus forcing it to pump more rapidly in an attempt to reduce the condition?

There must be a reason why my pulse is going down and I choose to think that a good sweat each day is part of it. By the sweat of thy brow shalt thou earn thy daily bread. Is this why farm workers are far less subject to heart disease than office-inhabiting men? Of course they exercise more, but I think it is the combination of the two. Exercise breaks down old cells, causing new ones to form. It gives rise to an increase in the flow of blood. Breathing is extended, and body functions stimulated. Muscles are kept in good repair, and their "tone" improved. There is a great improvement in the coordination of muscles and nerves. The circulation and eliminating processes of the body are stimulated.

If you want to see an example of a heart shouting for help, examine my pulse readings for July 12, 13 and 14. A few weeks later I am able to do the same walk without the pulse once going over 90. An hour a day of walking exercise must be a remarkable tonic to the body. I believe it is better than playing golf once or twice a week.

[304]

I was surprised, on August 1, 1954, to read in the Sunday *New York Times* magazine section that Roger Bannister, who recently broke the one-mile running record, was able to do so by a method he used of reducing his pulse. "By making his heart a more muscular pump, he was able to reduce his pulse beat from its original 72 in repose to below 50," says this magazine. By making his heart a more muscular pump! That must be what I am doing to mine.

I wonder, as I keep walking, from month to month and year to year, will my heart get bigger to cope with the additional activity? There are some interesting speculations on the size of the heart in the book *The Approach to Cardiology*, by Crighton Bramwell (Oxford University Press, 1951). Dr. Bramwell has found that all marathon runners have large hearts. But, he asks, "Are we justified in regarding this enlargement as entirely attributable to their training? In doing so may we not be putting the cart before the horse? The marathon runner needs a big heart. Doubtless his heart hypertrophies (enlarges) as the result of prolonged training, but it seems possible that there is another factor concerned. May it not be that men who happen to have hearts somewhat bigger than the average make the best marathon runners? They start life with a natural advantage. If this be so, it is not the marathon running that makes the heart big, but the big heart that makes the marathon runner. Another feature peculiar to the marathon runner is that his resting pulse-rate generally is well below 60. This enables him to

[305]

increase his cardiac output without an undue increase in heart-rate."

Dr. Bramwell says that animals who are very active have low pulses. "For example," says he, "the resting pulse-rate of the hare, an exceedingly athletic animal, is under 70, while that of its cousin, the rabbit, a sedentary creature, who never strays far from his burrow, is over 200 . . . To compensate for the difference in pulse rate, the hare's heart, relative to its body weight, is 3 times as large as the rabbit's."

But at a meeting of the Society of Physicians in Vienna, on June 8, 1956, Drs. Slapak and Prokep stated that enlargement of the heart may be found very frequently, but not universally, in athletes, and that it develops gradually in the course of years and depends on the kind of sport indulged in. Marathon running no doubt would produce it in most cases. In other words, a large heart moving slower is better than a small heart moving faster.

Dr. Joseph B. Wolffe, president of the College of Sports Medicine, recently said, "In runners over the age of 40 we found no clinical signs whatever of the onset of atherosclerosis, so common in middle life among the physically inactive . . . we are convinced, from our extensive studies, that the often blamed wear and tear of physical activity over prolonged years, far from hastening the so-called degenerative process associated with aging, actually prevents and inhibits disease." There is much evidence that exercise works some of the cholesterol out of the blood and artery walls.

There is a belief abroad that athletes suffer from

what is termed "athlete's heart." This is a myth and the *Journal of the American Medical Association* (See *Time*, July 26, 1954) advised that it is a condition that does not exist and that the term should be abolished. This article by Dr. Thomas K. Cureton of the Physical Fitness Research Laboratory, University of Illinois, stated that the reason why the health of some athletes deteriorates in middle age is not because of the activity of their athletic work in their youth, but because of the sedentary life they lapsed into when they got older, as well as heavy eating, drinking, smoking, etc.

In my case during this program of walking, my doctor examined my heart action and blood pressure once and sometimes twice a week and was quite satisfied with what he observed. Such examinations are advisable in all cases of persons who have heart conditions, and who desire to increase their physical activity the way I did. My doctor noticed that the action of my heart was definitely improved, and my heart murmur was all but eliminated. My blood pressure which, when I began, was about 135/85 came down to 120/70, a figure well nigh perfect for a young person of 20. I was 56 at the first reading, 59 at the second. It is still 120/70 because I have continued averaging a one-hour walk every day. Today I rarely suffer from my old time angina chest pressure symptoms.

Not every heart case will be permitted to do what I have done. The physician must be the judge in each case. There may be serious cases where extreme caution will be in order. There are damaged hearts, and those that have experienced thrombosis, occlusions and surgery. These persons must depend on their physicians for guidance.

A good method to inform you as to how you are reacting to the exercise, is to observe your ability to recuperate after it. Your heart should quiet itself in a minute or two. But if you are still breathing hard and your pulse has not come down in 7 or 8 minutes, it is a sign that you must exercise less.

Eventually, this walking program brought my "at rest" pulse down to 68. The other day I ran after a bus and was able to do it with the greatest of ease, whereas formerly there would have been an aftermath of pounding of the heart and breathlessness.

A few days ago I made a startling observation. My first heart symptoms had appeared in 1937, but it was in 1949 that they became really temperamental and troublesome. It was then that I increased my vitamin E dosage astronomically in order to relieve the chest pressure symptoms. Now I think I know the reason why. A friend and I used to go on hikes, sometimes for eight or nine miles. It was in 1949 that he moved to Philadelphia and from then on I fell into a most sedentary routine—no long walks; and my heart rebelled.

I was told recently of a man who for forty years was a track-walker for a railroad. For eight hours each day he walked the tracks to check for imperfections. A few years ago he retired and said, "Now I will rest." He then sat on his porch all day long. He was a healthy man, but within a year they laid him away to eternal rest. He had a heart attack. His heart could not stand the killing inactivity.

Recently I acquired an electrified indoor exercising

bicycle called the Exercycle upon which I sit for about one-half to three-quarters of an hour total per day, divided into about 3 sessions. I purchased this especially for use in inclement winter weather, but use it even though I walk my hour a day. I have already seen excellent results from it in stimulation of my circulation. The pedals turn fast by electricity and your feet have to move along with it. It is the equivalent of running. The seat moves up and down too, thus exercising the sacroiliac. This machine was highly recommended by my chiropractor. In fact, that is why I purchased it. If you are interested in the Exercycle, write to Exercycle Corporation, 630 Third Avenue, New York, N.Y. 10017.

I also acquired a rocking chair. What I want is as much movement as possible even when at rest. The rocking action is supposed to keep the fluid in the spine in movement and to be invigorating to the spinal nerves. Here is an interesting letter, regarding a rocking chair, received from a reader: "I have a friend who had a spinal operation of a serious type (the coccyx bone was cut from the spinal cord, leaving the spinal cord free). After a period of three months recuperation, she saw the doctor and had an examination and consultation with him. Her record of improvement was excellent and she asked the doctor what the next step was on her way to recovery. He told her that she should spend several hours a day in a rocking chair—not to the point of overtiring herself, but that she should rock daily. This, the doctor told her, would strengthen and help rejuvenate the nerves in her spine and get the spinal fluid working normally once more.

[309]

"She has been faithfully rocking ever since. When her many friends come to visit, they invariably will find her rocking away, and she sits and talks to them as she rocks. As a matter of fact, her friends tease her about it and call her the rocking chair lady, but she doesn't mind. This rocking is helping her to improve each day. (Her doctor is a brain and spine specialist in Florida.)"

I do not wish to overlook the fact that I also take setting-up exercises. This I have been doing ever since I was about 15 years old, when I bought the Swoboda system of how to be a success, which included a method of exercising.

I also wish to mention the fact that I have been getting some pointers in walking from a *Prevention* reader, Milton Feher of 200 W. 58th St. , New York, N.Y. Milton conducts a school of corrective exercising and general conditioning and has an excellent following in and around New York. He had written me that he was aware of how much walking I did, and was I aware that if I didn't walk right, I would be using up too much energy? As a result, on my periodic trips to New York, I drop in to see Milton and get a few pointers, not only in walking but also in various phases of exercising, body balance, etc. I must say that I've learned a few valuable things that I'll share with my readers later on. Mr. Feher is a former ballet dancer.

Recently I received a letter from a friend who said, "You looked wonderful the last time I saw you." (He hadn't seen me for several years.) "Your new 'walk a mile' regimen seems to do you good." It pays to walk. You get nice compliments.

My daughter Ruth writes me that in *The Adams*

[310]

Family, by James T. Adams, the author says that at Ghent during the peace arrangements of the War of 1812, "Adams usually went for a three hour walk, which appealed to none of his colleagues." He lived to be 81. I don't know how much his father used to walk, but he lived to be 91.

I can tell you another thing about walking. It is a great help in halitosis. I once knew a man who was a storekeeper and suffered horribly from this affliction for years. During the depression I ran into him on Broadway and he told me a sad tale of woe. He had lost his business and was unemployed, so he spent a lot of time in walking. I caught a whiff of his breath. It was like that of a newborn baby.

Another important advantage of walking is what it does to the specific gravity of the body. If you recall the chapter on specific gravity, you will admit that the specific gravity of my body must have improved greatly (increased) by this daily exercise. More research should be done on the effect of specific gravity and heart disease deaths. I believe a formula could be worked out in which the specific gravity, the pulse and the blood pressure of people could be computed mathematically and transformed into one figure, and by studying such figures in relation to the figure for people who have suffered a heart attack, a table could be produced showing safe values and danger points. This would be a money saving project for some insurance company. Certainly the insurance height and weight tables are ridiculously outmoded.

I have become so used to these walks that I would not know what to do without them. They give me an opportunity to think and to meditate. I carry little yellow pieces of paper in my pockets for note-taking on ideas that come to me during such periods and there is something about them that makes them come. Once, I counted over 30 separate notes taken during a one-hour period.

I would like to close this chapter with a reference on walking from the *Science News Letter* of July 21, 1956:

"The Greeks believed long walks are a good tonic for healthy living, according to Dr. Arthur Patch Mc-Kinlay, emeritus professor of Latin at the University of California at Los Angeles.

"Walking was described by the Greek (*sic*) writer, Pliny the Elder, as one of the 'Medicines of the Will,' he reports, explaining 'you have to have will power enough to take them.'

"Pliny was not writing as an expert but was merely passing on to his readers, the findings of prominent Greek physicians, one of whom was Hippocrates.

"Hippocrates mentions walking 40 times in one chapter on digestive diseases. He prescribes brisk walks, short walks, early morning walks, after-dinner walks, night walks.

"Early morning walks were recommended for emotional disturbances. Morning and evening walks for oversensitive persons. Brisk strolls to reduce hallucinations, reduce weight, and to keep the figure trim.

"Dr. McKinlay regularly takes a walk of from three to five miles daily. Still hale and hearty at 85, he has decided the Greeks were right when they described walking as one of the best forms of exercise in the world."

[312]

Part Eight:

HINTS ON CHOOSING THE RIGHT DIET

CHAPTER XXXVI

Regulate Fat Intake

One of the clearest and most sensible interpretations of the controversy over fats in the diet and their relation to heart and artery disease appeared in the *Royal Society of Health Journal* (England) for May-June, 1960. It was written by H. M. Sinclair of Oxford University, one of today's giants in nutrition research.

Dr. Sinclair begins by defining coronary heart disease. It is caused by the thickening of the walls of the blood vessel leading to the heart—the coronary artery. This is what doctors call atherosclerosis and we generally speak of as hardening of the arteries. It is not exactly "hardening." It involves the deposit of a "mush" of certain substances—fats, protein and minerals—on the inner wall of the artery. Such a thickening causes the narrowing in the passageway so that not enough blood reaches the heart. Medical terms used for various

[315]

aspects of this disease are ischemic heart disease, myocardial infarction, coronary heart disease, coronary thrombosis or heart attack.

The increase in the disease has been astonishingly rapid during the 20th Century. Dr. Sinclair quotes a noted physician of the past century who stated that he did not see a single case of this disease during 10 years of practice at a Montreal hospital. At present it is the commonest single cause of death in western countries. The apparent increase in deaths from heart disease in men in England and Wales, for instance, is nearly threefold since 1940. In 1921 the death rate from angina pectoris was 41, whereas in 1957 the rate was 2,209.

Studying the incidence of the disease in various countries, Dr. Sinclair tells us that many interesting facts come to light, none seeming to point to any one factor which is responsible. Why should the Japanese in Japan have a lower death rate from heart disease than Japanese in Hawaii? Why should Japanese living in California have a higher rate than those living in either Hawaii or Japan? Why should Mexico have the lowest death rate from heart disease, while France stands lower in the scale than the United States, England or Finland?

Looking for a nutritional cause of heart disease has preoccupied Dr. Sinclair for many years and he insists that the cause is dietary. The past few years have made almost every one of us aware of the word "cholesterol" used in conjunction with heart and artery disease. Cholesterol is a fatty substance which is an important part

[316]

of human cells. It is made in the body by various tissues; we do not have to get it in our food. But fatty foods of animal origin contain cholesterol.

We have known for a long time that in certain diseases the amount of cholesterol in the blood is increased: diabetes, deficiency in the thyroid gland and a kidney disease known as nephrosis. In these conditions hardening of the arteries and heart disease are unusually common. Carefully accumulated statistics show that men aged 40 to 60 who had a cholesterol level in their blood below 210 suffered only about half as many heart attacks as men whose levels were higher than 210. There seems to be good evidence, says Dr. Sinclair, that a high cholesterol level in the blood may indicate a susceptibility to heart attacks.

Another angle of the controversy over fats in the blood involves a different kind of fat—the unsaturated fatty acids. These are a kind of fat found most plentifully in vegetable and cereal foods. One of them, linoleic acid, is called an "essential" fatty acid, because it cannot be manufactured by the body, but must be supplied in the food we eat. Research seems to show that considerable animal fat in the diet (butter, cream and fat meat, for instance) increases one's need for linoleic acid. Also—and we think this point is very important— eating a great deal of carbohydrate (starchy or sweet) food from which the body can make the wrong kind of fats *increases the need in the diet for the essential ones.*

It sounds confusing, but actually all we are saying is that the more you eat of animal fats, the more you need of the other kind of fats—the ones found mostly

[317]

YOUR DIET AND YOUR HEART

in cereals and vegetables. So both aspects of diet are important—how much animal fat (and hence cholesterol) you get, and how much you get in *relation to how much you get of vegetable fats*. If you are a person who normally eats a diet very low in animal fats (no dairy products, no meat but very lean meat) and very low in starches (no desserts, no bread or other starches like macaroni and noodles) then you may need very little of the unsaturated fats to balance the amount of animal fats you get. But if you eat, as most Americans do, large amounts of animal fats, and/or large amounts of starchy foods, then it seems that you will need larger amounts of the unsaturated fats to balance the intake of those fats which are called "saturated."

Dr. Sinclair feels certain that this is the answer to hardening of the arteries and heart trouble—this important relationship between the two different kinds of fat in your diet. If there's not, in your blood, enough of the unsaturated fats, or if there is too much of the saturated ones, then the proper substances cannot be formed so that cholesterol can be absorbed properly into your tissues and it will accumulate. The accumulation of these cholesterol deposits occurs mostly in parts of the blood vessels which have been weakened by high blood pressure or undue strain—and sure enough, these are the areas especially subject to hardening of the arteries.

You will remember that we quoted earlier figures on heart disease among men. They are much higher among men than among women in younger age groups. In the light of such figures, it is interesting to find that the requirement for unsaturated fats (linoleic acid) is much greater among male laboratory animals than among females, during the earlier years of life. Does it not seem that this might be a very significant aspect of the problem?

Another angle—and we think this one is extremely important—Dr. Sinclair tells us that he has been doing some "preliminary work" experimenting with chlorine and mice. He has found that free chlorine can combine with the unsaturated fats, thus increasing the body's need for these essential ingredients of food. Does chlorinated water have the same effect? He feels that research is urgently needed. "It is possible, for instance," he says, "that one of the greatest public health measures ever introduced—the chlorination of public water supplies—could assist the disease." We know that chlorine destroys vitamin E as well. Is it not possible that drinking chlorinated water may make the city dweller more susceptible to heart disease than the country dweller? We know that the disease is far commoner in urban communities. We agree with Dr. Sinclair that research is urgently needed on this subject. No one has ever done any research on the possible effects of drinking chlorinated water over one's lifetime. This fact comes to us from the *Journal of the American Medical Association,* July 28, 1951. Isn't it about time we find out how much of our terrible heart disease mortality may be at least partly caused by chlorinated water?

Overweight and lack of exercise are two other certain causes of heart trouble, according to Dr. Sinclair. "Much evidence is available," he says, "that men who

[319]

are overweight tend to have higher mortality from coronary thrombosis than men who are underweight." The danger may lie in the process of *becoming* fat, Dr. Sinclair believes. One researcher has found that, if exercise is sufficient to prevent weight gain, diets high in calories and fat can be fed without increasing the blood cholesterol levels. So exercise and overweight and cholesterol levels are closely related. If you eat too much, especially of fat and starches, and get too little exercise, you are more likely to have too much cholesterol in the blood. If you eat and exercise moderately there is less chance. And even if you eat more than you should, but don't put on weight because you "work" it off with exercise, your cholesterol level will probably remain low. Perhaps this may be another reason why country folks have less heart disease than urban folks. Even with today's mechanized farming, country people surely get more physical exercise than city people.

McDonald and Fullerton, writing in *The Lancet*, volume ii, page 600, tell us that high-fat meals cause the blood to coagulate more rapidly. This might explain a number of heart attacks and "strokes" caused by blood clots. However, these two researchers found that moderate physical exercise abolished this threat. The blood did not coagulate too rapidly in those who exercised.

Another angle to the heart disease problem is smoking. Dr. Sinclair tells us that there is no doubt there are more deaths from heart disease in men of 45 to 62 among those who smoke than among those who do not

[320]

smoke. The levels of cholesterol in the blood are also higher in smokers. Interestingly enough, one investigator has found that smokers consume more fat in their diets than non-smokers! This may play some part in the picture.

What about "stress"? Do we have more heart attacks because we are living at a faster pace than we used to? Investigators have found that, during periods of stress, the blood cholesterol level rises. Students tested just before examinations, soldiers tested during periods of stress, have been found to have high cholesterol levels during such times. So, during periods of personal stress, one should take special pains to eat healthfully and exercise faithfully. So far as today's "pace" is concerned, Editor Rodale has shown in his book *This Pace Is Not Killing Us* that we actually live much more easily today than at any time in the past.

To return to Dr. Sinclair's basic theory, he believes that the most important factor of all to be considered in heart disease is diet and the most significant item in the diet is its fat. There is still plenty of controversy among nutrition experts as to which kind of fat does the damage. A famous American researcher, Ancel Keys, believes that the total amount of fat in the diet is the important thing. All fats in the diet raise the level of cholesterol in the blood, says he. But, says Dr. Sinclair, other researchers have shown that vegetable fats (salad oils, nuts, seeds, avocados) tend to lower blood cholesterol, while animal fats raise it. In addition, they have found that some vegetable fats raise

[321]

cholesterol and others lower it, while some fats from fish (fish liver oils and food fish that is fatty) lower the cholesterol level. So it seems that the secret of which kind of fat has a beneficial effect on the cholesterol level involves the unsaturated fatty acids. Those foods which contain it (most vegetable and cereal seeds and oils and the fats from fish) lower cholesterol. Fats from animal sources (low in the unsaturated fatty acids) and a few rare fats among vegetable foods raise the cholesterol level.

Finally, the research done up to now seems to show that the important thing for heart and blood vessel health is not how much or how little of either kind of fat you get—but how much of the vegetable fat you get *in relation to how much of the animal fat you get.* The more animal fat you eat, the more vegetable fat you need. The less animal fat you eat the less vegetable fat you need.

An additional finding is that starches and sugars in your diet can be changed into the wrong kind of fat and hence, if you eat lots of these foods, you need more vegetable fats to balance the other fats. It is well to keep in mind too that the hydrogenation of fats destroys the valuable fatty acids. Hydrogenating fats makes them solid at room temperatures. Margarine contains hydrogenated fats. Most commercially sold peanut butter contains some hydrogenated fat; modern lard has been hydrogenated.

So far as processed foods are concerned, all of these probably contain harmful fats—prepared mixes, prepared foods like frozen fried food, pies, pastries, salted

[322]

nuts, crackers, pretzels—most of the foods most of us eat every day have been made using the wrong kind of fats.

What kind of fats shall we use? How about lard—isn't it as natural a fat as you can get? When vegetable fats are refined isn't their food value largely destroyed just as the food value of other refined foods suffers? How does olive oil compare to corn oil from the nutritional point of view?

First, let's talk about what we mean by "fats" in the diet. There are two kinds of fats—those that are solid at room temperature and those that are liquid. The liquid ones are generally spoken of as oils; the solid ones as fats. Of course all of them will become liquids at some high temperature (different in every case) and all liquid oils will become solids at low temperatures.

Fats and oils make up about 2 to 5 per cent of the average diet by weight. In many recent articles about fats we hear of the fat content of the American diet being as high as 40 per cent. We should keep in mind that this means that 40 per cent of the *calories* of the diet are from fat—not 40 per cent of the actual food eaten. Fat is high in calories, of course, so just a little fat adds considerably to this percentage.

Animal fats—all of them, including milk, butter, fat meats, lard, and so forth—contain cholesterol, the substance that apparently constitutes a grave danger to us since it appears to be responsible for hardening of the arteries, heart disease, gallstones and so forth. Vegetable fats contain no cholesterol. To take its place they have sitosterols, which do not act the same way.

[323]

Vegetable fat contains, too, what we call unsaturated fatty acids, as opposed to the saturated fatty acids that are contained in greater quantity in foods of animal origin. Although there is still considerable debate over the digestibility of fatty foods, we know for certain that the vegetable fats are more easily digested than the animal fats.

Lard, of course, comes from hog fat, hence contains cholesterol and lacks the useful fatty acids. Processors have, in recent years, been doing a lot of things to lard that make it even more objectionable as food. In an attempt to produce lard that compares with the vegetable shortening, they have added chemicals to prevent the lard from becoming rancid; they have hydrogenated and deodorized it.

Margarine is made from vegetable fats which have been hydrogenated. That is, hydrogen has been forced through them to produce a chemical change that makes the liquid oils solid, as margarine is. Such oils as cottonseed, soybean and, in Europe, whale oil, are used. Most margarine in this country is "fortified" with synthetic vitamin A. The reason is that the oils themselves contain very little vitamin A in comparison with butter.

We do not recommend using margarine, mostly because of the many chemical substances used in it, of which the synthetic vitamin A is only one. Artificial coloring, preservatives and so forth are also used. But in addition, hydrogenating the oils to make them solid destroys most of the essential fatty acids which are the chief reason for eating vegetable oils. So margarine is little better than butter as a spread, in spite of the fact

[324]

that it is made from substances that do not contain cholesterol.

Linseed oil (made from flaxseed), sardine and other fish oils are generally considered to be inferior for eating purposes, because of taste, even though they contain large amounts of unsaturated fatty acids.

Soybean oil is another popular vegetable oil. We are told that it presents some difficulties since it is subject to some slight "flavor reversion." We assume this means that its taste may suffer with age. Crude soybean oil is our best source of lecithin at present. Lecithin is the substance rich in unsaturated fatty acids which occurs in vegetable fats.

Sunflower seed oil, corn oil and poppyseed oil are all quite similar. Corn oil is a little darker in color than the others.

Cottonseed oil is the "standard American all-purpose edible oil," according to Jacobs in his book *Food and Food Products*, published by Interscience, 1951.

Peanut oil is suitable for all purposes for which cottonseed oil is used, except that it tends to cloud and thicken at low temperatures.

Rapeseed oil (we have never heard of this being used in this country), is difficult to deodorize and has an unpleasant reversion of flavor.

Olive oil is the most popular edible oil of Southern Europe and the Mediterranean. Its content of unsaturated fatty acids is not high, however. And we must watch out for the unsaturated fatty acid content of oils. It is important.

Olive oil is not treated to remove its taste and odor.

[325]

For this reason some folks feel that olive oil is far superior to other oils, "because it has such a marvelous taste," they say. Others, used to the bland salad oils that have been deodorized, cannot stand the taste or smell of olive oil. It is well to remember, when you are deciding among vegetable and seed oils, that olive oil is low in the unsaturated fatty acids—those extremely valuable substances so powerful for good in the way your body uses fat. On the other hand, it is unrefined which is a recommendation for it, we believe.

Corn oil has been used for extensive laboratory experiments. Much of what we know about the relation of cholesterol, lecithin, unsaturated fatty acids, vegetable and animal fats has been discovered in laboratories using corn oil as the source of unsaturated fatty acids in the diet of the laboratory animals.

An excellent book has been written by Dorothy M. Rathmann, Ph.D., entitled *Vegetable Oils in Nutrition, with special reference to unsaturated fatty acids*. The booklet is published by Corn Products Refining Company, 17 Battery Place, New York, N.Y. It is a technical book written for professional men—doctors, nutritionists and therapists.

Dr. Rathmann tells us, "The opinion is becoming more and more wide-spread that unsaturated vegetable oils, such as Mazola brand corn oil, possess distinct nutritional advantages. For example, the fact that diets containing corn oil result in lower serum cholesterol levels than do those containing more highly saturated fats has led to the hope that the incidence and

[326]

course of atherosclerosis may be influenced favorably, in part at least, by dietary means.

"This favorable effect of corn oil has been attributed to the presence of two different types of compounds capable of lowering serum cholesterol levels, namely sitosterols and essential fatty acids. In addition to a relationship to cholesterol metabolism the essential fatty acids also appear to have important functions in the development of new cells and the maintenance of healthy body tissues, particularly the skin, liver and kidneys. Requirements for the essential fatty acids seem to be increased when food yields large amounts of saturated or isomeric fatty acids, as may be the case in American diets rich in animal and hydrogenated vegetable fats."

The book contains a great deal of detailed information about experiments involving corn oil in relation to cholesterol deposits. The further information is given that corn oil contains: 53 per cent linoleic acid (the most important of the unsaturated fatty acids), 1.5 per cent of sitosterols and, of course, no cholesterol. Compare this to other fats containing unsaturated fatty acids:

Linoleic acid

Linseed oil	20 per cent
Sardine	15
Safflower	70
Poppyseed	62
Soybean	53
Sunflower	57

[327]

Sesame	41
Cottonseed	50
Rice bran	34
Peanut oil	25
Olive	8
Wheat germ	50
Corn	53

Corn oil is also high in linolenic acid and other fatty acids.

Our final suggestions to you, then, are these: Judging from the amount of information we have up to now we would counsel readers to avoid animal fats as much as possible, with the exception of eggs.

One cannot help getting some fat in meat, of course. But eliminate gravies and fatty sauces! Avoid butter and milk. Shun like poison the hydrogenated fats in which the important fatty acids have been destroyed. This means don't buy the white solid shortenings. And don't buy prepared, processed foods for you can be sure hydrogenated shortenings were used in them.

Do take wheat germ oil every day, because of its essential fatty acid content, vitamin E and the many other factors that it contains. For fats in your meals use salad oils—olive oil, if you like the taste (but remember it's low in the important fatty acids), corn oil, cottonseed oil—any of the salad oils you find at your grocery store.

Although many of the experiments quoted in the newspapers and in this article concern corn oil, this is simply because that happened to be the oil used by the researchers. It does not mean that other vegetable and cereal oils would be less effective in these same experiments.

We especially want to commend sunflower seed oil. As you see in the chart above, it is higher in linoleic acid than corn oil. And linoleic acid is generally credited as being the Good Fairy among the fatty acids which put unwanted cholesterol to flight. We are told that in unsaturated fatty acids as a whole, sunflower seed oil is higher than any other. Its vitamin E content, too, is extremely high—222 milligrams per hundred grams, compared to only 5 milligrams in sesame oil and 22 to 48 in peanut oil.

One of the articles which sparked the whole recent investigation of fats and oils in the diet was published in *The Lancet* for April 28, 1956. In this article a now classic experiment was described by Dr. Bronte-Stewart and his associates in which sunflower seed oil was one of those used to bring about a rapid decrease in blood cholesterol.

And remember, it seems to be true that the more of the processed fats you eat and the more animal fats you eat, the more you need of the vegetable fats, whose unsaturated fatty acids will counteract any cholesterol-forming tendency of the processed and animal fats, low in unsaturated fatty acids.

[329]

CHAPTER XXXVII

Special Dangers in Butterfat

There are many question marks and contradictions in the results of research on the relationship between diet and the level of serum cholesterol. Cholesterol is a perfectly natural type of fat that all mammalian animals including man synthesize within their own bodies because it is needed. It is one of the two body fats that are transformed into vitamin D by the action of sunlight. It is part of the material that sheathes and protects the nerves, and cholesterol has many other vital functions as well. It only becomes a problem when the amount of it in the blood stream becomes greater than 250 milligrams for every 100 milliliters of blood (250 mg. per cent). When the blood contains excessive amounts, cholesterol tends to combine with other blood elements into clots that can stick to the walls of arteries and thus narrow the blood passages or that can flow to the heart and damage it directly.

Because this much is known beyond dispute about blood cholesterol, many doctors have gotten into the precautionary habit of advising their patients to reduce the amount of cholesterol-containing foods in their diets. As more and more studies reach maturity, however, it becomes increasingly evident that *Prevention* has been absolutely right in advising its readers for many years that dietary cholesterol is not the cause of high serum cholesterol. One of the most important of these studies was reported in April, 1965, to the Annual Meeting of the Federation of American Societies for Experimental Biology.

Dr. D. Mark Hegsted, Ph.D., of the Harvard School of Public Health reported on a series of studies which showed that consuming from 22 per cent to 44 per cent of the total calories as fat, much of it high in cholesterol, does not necessarily have any influence on serum cholesterol levels. What *was* found to raise the cholesterol level was not cholesterol, but two fatty acids, the more active and important of which is known as myristic acid.

As reported in *Medical World News* (May 14, 1965), "Dr. Hegsted's team divided hospitalized men into two dietary groups. One group was placed on a low-fat diet, with 22 per cent of the calories supplied by fat. The other group received a high-fat diet, in which fat accounted for 38 per cent of the calories. The basic diet for both groups contained low-fat foods, and the total calories were made up by a variety of oils, which were changed at four-week intervals for test purposes. The cholesterol content of the diet, supplied

[331]

from egg yolk, was also varied. Test oils, including coconut, olive, safflower, cotton seed, corn, and fish oils, and butterfat, were added to the low-fat foods either singly or in combinations."

And what Dr. Hegsted found was that of the test fats enumerated above, it was the butterfat that played the most active role in raising serum cholesterol. This, he discovered, was due primarily to its high content of myristic acid and to a much lesser extent to palmitic acid. Egg yolk, which is so rich in cholesterol it is the basic material of cholesterol experiments, had no particular effect in raising serum cholesterol values.

This throws new light on how modern food production methods, geared only to the market without thought of the ultimate effect on health, may unwittingly be producing more heart attacks.

For one of the outstanding efforts of modern meat production has been to produce meat that contains more myristic acid. Why? Because myristic acid—the same myristic acid that has been found the true culprit in the dangerous effect some fats have on serum cholesterol—is the fatty acid that stiffens and solidifies meat fat and makes it whiter in color.

One of the best indications of this is a symposium on food quality published by the American Association for the Advancement of Science. In it A. M. Pearson of the Department of Food Science of Michigan State University points out, among other things, that such animal foods as "soybeans, peanuts, rice bran, rice polish, and chufas all produce soft pork, if fed in considerable amounts to the pig. Lard from soft hogs

[332]

does not harden at ordinary room temperature. The bacon is soft, flabby, and difficult to slice. On curing, the cuts have a much greater shrinkage, and cooking losses are greater than for pork from firm hogs. . . . Since the pig tends to produce a sufficiently hard fat from carbohydrate feeds, use of high-carbohydrate diets with elimination of soft, oily feeds results in production of firm pork." This firmness, of course, is produced by increasing the myristic acid content of the pork fat. In another point in the same paper, it is pointed out that the myristic acid in beef fat can also be increased by feeding grain containing 10 per cent animal fat.

It can thus be seen that it is not just a matter of money-hungry meat packers or cattlemen, but that even the food scientists of the universities think of improving the quality of food in terms of making it more attractive in appearance and handling qualities without bothering to find out what this may do to its nutritional value. They are not setting out to cause heart attacks. They are merely ignoring the entire question as irrelevant and it is this kind of neglect that manages to negate the advances in medicine so that neither longevity nor mortality rates show any substantial improvement.

A strong indictment of modern meat production methods is made by Arthur Blumenfeld in his book, *Heart Attack: Are You a Candidate?* (Paul S. Eriksson, New York). Blumenfeld contrasts the modern artificial diet of food animals with the former free-range diet, and finds an enormous and significant difference.

[333]

Writing of the old-fashioned methods of grazing cattle on the grassy plains, Blumenfeld says, "They wholly ate grass and slowly grew into marketable animals. But greater profits could be made if the animals exercised less and were fed more efficiently on corn and other grain spiked with chemical stimulants." He goes on to explain that the fat of the old-fashioned grass-fed cattle was yellowish in color, soft in texture, and that a significant proportion of it was unsaturated.

He points out that, in the old days when hogs used to root for their food on the free range, scientists used to use lard as an excellent source of unsaturated fats for their laboratory experiments. That is no longer possible. The fat we see on pork today is practically as hard and white as the beef fat, which phenomenon is brought about by a diet that increases the amount of myristic acid. And thus, the meat raisers have unwittingly been contributing to the increasing incidence of atherosclerosis.

It should be noted that while myristic acid (and to a lesser degree palmitic acid) have been incriminated as the cholesterol-raising elements in fat, this does not mean nor is it claimed that these are the only dietary reasons for high serum cholesterol. Dr. Hegsted was careful to point out in his Experimental Biology Federation paper that while fats are important, no single substance can be named as being entirely responsible for atherosclerosis. And we have already emphasized to our readers that another common food has been found to be even more dangerous. That food is common table sugar. Dr. John Yudkin, Professor of Nutrition

[334]

at the University of London, published a remarkable series of papers in *The Lancet* during the summer of 1964 in which he explored this question and showed by statistical studies made in London hospitals that almost invariably, the patient with atherosclerosis consumes twice as much sugar as those of equivalent age, weight and living conditions who are free of atherosclerosis. Since it was also discovered last year that cholesterol is manufactured in the liver directly from acetic acid, which is a degradation product of the digestion of sugar, the connection is obvious.

It becomes more and more apparent than in the dietary, the way to avoid atherosclerosis is to eliminate sugar and dairy products from the diet and be very sparing about the amount of meat fat that is consumed. On the positive side, you can help hold down your serum cholesterol with a diet rich in all the vitamins and minerals and an emphasis on lean meats and raw fruits and vegetables. Vitamins C and B complex, the polyunsaturated fats such as we get from egg yolk, soybeans and corn, and the pectin from fruits and vegetables have all been shown to have a cholesterol-lowering effect. In addition, probably the best guarantee of a normal cholesterol metabolism is a healthfully functioning liver. And you cannot name a single nutrient that is not in some way connected with the health of the liver.

[335]

CHAPTER XXXVIII

Beans for Better Hearts

Are you, like most people, confused over the best
diet to follow to try to prevent coronary heart disease,
the leading killer disease of our day? Well, if you are,
take hope, because it looks like a sound dietary prevention plan is finally emerging from what we might
call the "cholesterol chaos." A new heart diet plan is
being drawn up by some of the country's best scientists,
and the public will be surprised to find that some of
the foods we thought in the past to be among the most
healthful will be on the banned list. And other foods
that have been scorned as too cheap and unglamorous
to pay much attention to will likely become a very large
part of our day-to-day diet.

Cholesterol control will still be partly the purpose
of the new heart health diet, but the main object will
be to seek a balance of a whole range of biochemical

[336]

alterations, primarily through the eating of the proper kinds and amounts of carbohydrates. You will soon be reading of and hearing a lot more about "simple" carbohydrates as opposed to "complex" carbohydrates, and those two terms may hold the key to a level of heart health which is now far beyond the reach of most Americans. It isn't too soon to start preparing ourselves now for this new type of diet.

Let's back-track to cholesterol for a moment. The early discoveries that people with coronary artery and heart disease had more than average cholesterol in their blood were momentous, as were the findings that certain foods (particularly saturated fats) seemed to be associated with high blood cholesterol levels. Unfortunately, those findings were so impressive to both scientists and the public that they were over-exploited in many ways. Scientists inclined to study the heart-diet link concentrated on the fat-cholesterol link, to the exclusion of other possible leads. Those who didn't want to believe that coronary disease and diet could be related went to work to demolish the cholesterol theory. Investigation of other fruitful heart-diet links was therefore delayed by overconcentration on cholesterol.

That situation has now been changed to a degree by scientists who recognized some years back that coronary heart disease was an illness caused by many factors of which diet was only one. And there was a group of scientists within that large group who suspected—perhaps were convinced—that cholesterol was itself not

[337]

the most promising lead to follow for an answer to the diet-heart question. They still recognize cholesterol as a valued indicator of artery health, but feel that other substances—particularly the triglycerides—are more likely to be the most important blood factor to watch, and to try to influence through diet changes. And they are turning the spotlight not on fats in the diet, but on carbohydrates, which are being segregated into good (complex) carbohydrates and bad (simple) carbohydrates. I will give you more explanation of that intriguing separation later, but it might help to keep in mind the rough guide that sugars are simple carbohydrates and starchy foods tend to be high in complex carbohydrates.

The American Medical Association recognized the importance of carbohydrate nutrition and metabolism to coronary heart disease control in an editorial in the September 25 issue of its *Journal.*

Three main points were made:

1. A single diet plan won't suffice to provide best coronary disease prevention in all people. However, it was pointed out that 90 per cent of the experimental subjects observed by Dr. P. T. Kuo, a leading investigator of the carbohydrate-heart link, reacted very favorably to a diet low in simple carbohydrates and high in complex carbohydrates. The *JAMA* article noted that "Kuo's data indicate that sensitivity to simple carbohydrate is widespread among both healthy and atherosclerotic populations in America."

2. Although there are still gaps in our present knowledge, the AMA noted that triglycerides and carbohy-

[338]

drate metabolism have a fundamental role as diet factors involved in the cause of coronary disease.

3. It is now up to physicians to find out which of their patients in the high-risk coronary disease group react unfavorably to a high fat diet, which are sensitive to carbohydrates of the wrong sort, and which people may be being led to increased heart risk by both of those dietary factors.

John Yudkin, an imaginative English physician-researcher, led the way into the carbohydrate-heart field with his revelation that consumption of sugar (simple carbohydrate) usually is closely associated with consumption of saturated fats. He challenged the logic of previous statistical studies which showed a link between saturated fats, cholesterol and coronary disease. Yudkin said that the assumption that saturated fats started the chain of events could well be false. His figures showed that as people increased their intake of fats, they ate more sugar too—and it was his belief that the sugar is doing most of the harm.

Laboratory backing for Yudkin's theory has come recently from Dr. P. T. Kuo of the University of Pennsylvania. It was that work which spurred the editors of the *Journal of the American Medical Association* to write their September 25 editorial, telling doctors to start finding out which patients who are candidates for heart attacks might be reacting unfavorably to refined carbohydrates in their diet.

The evidence against refined sugar (simple carbohydrates) now seems almost airtight. Less well proven but perhaps equally intriguing is the idea that some of

[339]

the complex carbohydrates—the starchy foods—may be as good for you as sugar is bad. And nutritionists are pointing out that there are other simple carbohydrates besides refined sugar. All sugars are simple carbohydrates, including the sugar in such natural foods as honey and fruits. Potatoes are the one vegetable whose carbohydrate is largely in starch form, and therefore potatoes rank solidly on the complex carbohydrate list along with other starchy foods like corn, beans and cereals.

Seeing fruits on a list of foods that are thought to be harmful to many people (because of their simple carbohydrate content) is a shocker. Health-minded people have long ostracized white sugar as a non-healthful food, but to think that the sugar in an apple or a peach can be just as bad is indeed startling. Not only is it a difficult idea for the diet-minded community to accept, but it is an idea which the orthodox nutritionists are fiddling with at arm's length too. Perhaps that is why we have read so little about it in the popular press, which tries to be several jumps ahead of the more proven concepts that appear in the professional journals.

We are not ready, by any means, to say or even imply that sweet tasting natural foods are now on the suspect list just because they contain simple carbohydrates. Such foods are an extremely important source of vitamins and minerals for many people and to eliminate them from the diet just because the doctors have come up with a new theory about food and heart disease would be foolhardy. Who knows what the

[340]

How can nature think?

doctors will be recommending a few years from now? However, we should learn all we can about these new theories as they are born, and should be ready to put to use new knowledge about nutrition when we can really be sure that what is new is also what is right.

Our own inclination, of course, is always to relate new nutritional ideas to the concept that foods in their natural state are best because they are whole, unrefined, and are therefore likely to contain all the food elements which nature thought necessary to put in that food. We have seen often in the past how that theory has proved true in the long run, while medical diet fashions come and go. Of course, there are some toxins that occur naturally in certain foods, like moulds which grow when some seeds are stored improperly, but they are extremely rare.

However, the good case that has been made out against simple carbohydrates—even in certain whole, natural foods—might cause us to add a new criterion to our evaluation of how natural a food is. Perhaps we should add the dimensions of time and quantity as well as quality to our equation. For example, a food like the apple is certainly natural, but to a primitive man an apple was available for eating only a short time of the year. Therefore, we might ask ourselves whether we are being natural in eating a lot of apples all year long, even if they are unsprayed and organically grown. While we don't want to equate ourselves with primitive man, we have to recognize that people in the past got along for millions of years on diets that are very different from what we are now eating. We would

[341]

be foolish to ignore completely the historical perspective of diet, at least for purposes of comparison.

What did primitive man eat, you might ask? The answer is that he lived mainly on seeds and tubers that he collected, which could be stored for long periods. Seeds and tubers are, of course, prime sources of complex carbohydrates. So are legumes, which he probably ate in liberal amounts. He also ate meat (animal protein and saturated fat) when he could kill game, and fish. Simple carbohydrates were the exception and not the rule in his diet, primarily because they were available to him only in foods that came along only for brief periods.

We are not suggesting that we immediately change our eating habits to avoid all simple carbohydrates, even if they come to us in natural foods. We can cut down drastically on simple carbohydrates by not eating refined sugar, which accounts for about 20 per cent of *all* carbohydrates in the diet of most people. It could be that those people who are found by medical tests to have high levels of triglycerides in their blood will soon be advised to stay away from all simple carbohydrates. Perhaps what the average person should do now is learn more about the different types of carbohydrates and try to eat more complex carbohydrate foods as a substitute for foods containing refined sugar. There can be no medical argument against the logic of such a plan. Carbohydrates have been an unfashionable food component for a number of years, primarily becauce of their reputation as fat producers. But we do need carbohydrates for energy, and there is no

[342]

reason why we should shy away from a reasonable amount of complex carbohydrate foods.

Dried beans are a useful and tasty food which seems to meet all of the current requirements for heart health. They are free of saturated fat and rich in protein and complex carbohydrates. Not only that but they are one of the cheapest foods you can buy, easily stored, flavorful, and work right into a number of good recipes. In 1965 in the *Journal of Nutrition,* Drs. Grande, Anderson and Keys reported that when bread and potatoes were substituted for sucrose (sugar, simple carbohydrate) in the diet of men, no lowering of cholesterol was reported. But when leguminous seeds (beans) were the source of complex carbohydrates, cholesterol levels did drop. In fact, Ancel Keys has become so enamoured of the health virtues of beans that he and his wife have written a fine little cookbook called *The Benevolent Bean.*

In their new book, *The Benevolent Bean,* (Doubleday and Co., Inc.) the authors describe studies which to their surprise suggest a strong link between the low coronary heart disease in Italy and the Italians' love of beans. They began their investigation right at the source: They checked into the University of Naples.

It was apparent almost at once that the Neapolitans live on a generally low-fat diet—only 20 to 25 per cent of the total daily calories are provided by fats, compared with 35 per cent in England and 40 per cent in Minnesota. The only segment of the Neapolitan population with any heart problem to speak of was the small upper-crust set, who ate a richer diet than most

[343]

natives can afford. These few were plagued by the same circulatory problems as their English and American cousins. This enabled the Keys to conclude that the Neapolitans had basically the same constitution as the English and American men in the observation groups. But what was different about the ordinary Neapolitan's way of life?

To find out, an experiment was set up involving 24 physically healthy Minnesotans who ate first an ordinary American diet and then a diet matching that of Naples in the percentage of fat, protein and carbohydrate calories for a pre-determined period. As expected, the cholesterol readings fell from 225 to 195 when a low fat diet was introduced. But 195 was still far above the average Neapolitan figure of 165.

Well, in truth, Minnesota was not using a real Neapolitan diet. Certainly the fat, protein and carbohydrates were matched, the minerals and vitamins were adequate and similar and the calorie balance was also maintained; but there were differences in the actual foods the experimental subjects were eating. Neapolitans get their fat chiefly from olive oil; the Minnesota group got its fat from meat and milk. This observation ties in with the work of Dr. Lawrence Kinsell in California who found that vegetable oils substituted in equal amounts for common hard fats in the diet can predictably cut cholesterol levels. On the strength of this work, the data from the Minnesota experiment with the improper fat was recalculated. But the cholesterol values in Naples were still 10 to 15 per cent lower than could be explained by the fats in the diet.

[344]

What else was there about the Neapolitan diet? "Where were the mountains of leafy vegetables, the abundant fruits, the beans and other leguminous seeds, so prominent in the daily diet of Naples?" asks Dr. Keys. New experiments were set up, this time using regular Neapolitan fare. The differences in serum cholesterol levels between the Neapolitans and the Minnesota men all but disappeared.

The next question: what particular thing is there in the beans, vegetables, and fruits of Naples that doesn't appear in the bread and potatoes that usually take their place in the American diet?

Menus were compared once more in particular detail. One item stood out: the difference in the amount of beans in the diets. Americans eat far fewer beans than Neapolitans. In Italy pasta and beans (pasta e fagioli) appears regularly in the diet of most ordinary Italians, about once a week.

A new test was set up. This time a group of men were kept on a regular diet, except for periods when beans replaced equal calories of simple carbohydrates (potatoes, sugar and lactose). Another group of men made the reverse replacement, using carbohydrates instead of beans. The serum cholesterol went down about 9 per cent when the men were eating beans compared with the reading when beans were replaced by a bean protein and simple carbohydrate.

So there it was. The effect of beans on the diet has been proven, and the result was confirmed with experiments using brown beans in Holland and chick-peas in India. "So if you happen to be interested in cholesterol

[345]

control," says Keys, "beans, or any leguminous seeds merit a prominent place in our diet."

If you take Dr. Keys' advice you have over 10,000 species of beans to choose from. But practically speaking, there are only about a dozen kinds readily available in the U.S. Almost all leguminous seeds are edible, but preparation of some species is so complicated and troublesome that they are ignored by all but the most avid bean eaters.

We are not big bean consumers. Department of Agriculture estimates show that the average American puts away only about 7.5 pounds of dried beans and peas a year. And this figure includes peanuts, which Americans gobble at the rate of 5 pounds a year per person. The 2.5 pounds that are left of the 7.5 clearly demonstrates that Americans can't be accused of overindulging in beans.

To help you set a safe, but worthwhile quota for yourself, consider Dr. Keys' report on experimental subjects who ate 100 grams (over 3 ounces) of beans a day for months and had no problem; in one district of southern Italy the average person eats 82 grams of beans a day as part of his customary menu. If Americans ate only a half pound of beans a week it would double our intake of legumes.

If we did that, Dr. Keys suggests, "Something else in the diet would have to be reduced to keep total calories in line. Our proposal would be to reduce sugar. Nutritionally and gastronomically too, it is scandalous that Americans get some 16 per cent of their calories from sugar and other sweeteners. If we substituted 12

[346]

pounds of beans for an equal amount of sugar in the yearly diet, we would still be eating around 85 pounds of sugar a year."

Nutritionally speaking, beans are an excellent addition to any menu. They contain appreciable amounts of calcium, phosphorus and iron along with vitamins B_1 and B_2, niacin, and to a lesser degree vitamin C. Of course they are rich in protein. Concerning the quality of the protein in beans, Dr. Keys writes, "Protein quality is evaluated in various ways, most commonly by measuring the weight growth of young rats fed on a diet containing the test protein. . . . With such experiments in which the test protein is the only protein in the diet, soybean protein turns out to have a little lower quality than beef muscle protein, but the protein of peas or ordinary beans may be only 60 per cent as good as the meat protein. . . . But this is not a realistic approach: no one has only one kind of protein in the diet. A combination of bean and cereal protein is nearly as efficient as meat protein. Many populations the world over actually have developed smart answers to the protein problem this way. . . ."

If it's fat you want to cut down on in the diet, beans are made to order. Most beans contain less than 2 per cent fat, and the fat they do contain is not only low in saturated fats, it is high in the essential fatty acid, linoleic acid (desirable) and tends to be very high in linolenic acid (also desirable).

We humans have been in the bean business for thousands, perhaps millions of years. Scientists have uncovered evidence that legumes were cultivated back

[347]

in the Neolithic Period, when man first entered the stage of food producing. Lentils were piled in Egyptian tombs of the 12th Dynasty (2400-2200 B.C.). The Bible mentions that Jacob gave Esau "bread and pottage of lentils." Beans are mentioned by nearly every explorer of the Americas from Columbus on.

Now is a good time for you to discover, or rediscover, beans in your own kitchen for your own good health.

[348]

CHAPTER XXXIX

More Value in Organic Foods

What is the leading cause of heart attacks? Ask any-one—your doctor, your bus driver, your secretary. You'll get the same answer. Cholesterol—which causes atherosclerosis, which leads to formation of a clot which shuts off circulation to the heart.

There is only one thing wrong with this commonly held belief. Mounting medical evidence, recently sum-marized by Dr. P. Prioreschi in the *Canadian Medical Association Journal* (April 29, 1967), strongly indi-cates that it just isn't so.

Dr. Prioreschi, a Canadian doctor, reviewed the re-sults of experiments conducted by many investigators all over the world to advance the new concept that myocardial infarction (death of some of the heart muscle tissue) is not due to a thrombotic occlusion of a coronary artery but rather to a metabolic derangement in the tissue. "In fact," says Dr. Prioreschi, "The coronary circulation did not seem to play a very important role in the development of the lesions."

Granted that the atherosclerosis is at times an accessory to the crime because this condition slows down circulation to the heart and therefore may favor the formation of necrotic (dead or dying) tissue. But, according to evidence coming to seem increasingly important, it is the death of some of the heart cells that causes heart attacks, rather than being caused by the attacks as had formerly been believed. And it is a metabolic derangement that causes the tissue cells to die.

And the really exciting news that comes out of Dr. Prioreschi's report pertains to the role of potassium in the prevention of cardiac necroses.

In a large variety of papers cited by Dr. Prioreschi, it has been well established that a number of substances widely found in our environment are actively toxic to the heart and can be used experimentally to induce heart attacks. Most important and most frightening is sodium chloride (common table salt) which is not only used everywhere but is also packed into just about every commercially processed food a person can buy—even baby foods. Other cardio-toxic agents were commonly used drugs—aureomycin, polymyxin and cortisone. Obviously anything toxic to the tissues of the heart should be avoided if possible.

Even more impressive than the listing of cardiotoxins which might number into the thousands if every possibility were investigated, was the discovery that one

[350]

MORE VALUE IN ORGANIC FOODS

particular mineral nutrient was able in almost every case to counteract their effects and prevent heart attacks. That mineral is potassium.

The information gained by this study will no doubt find its way into accepted medical practice. But the time lag from test tube to table is anywhere from ten to thirty years.

By applying these findings now to improve our own nutrition, we have the power in our own hands to shorten that gap and enhance our chances for good healthy hearts—in our time.

Since sodium was one of the main cardiotoxic agents used in the experiments—the very first step would be to throw away that salt shaker. While your body needs some sodium, there is so much of it in commercially prepared foods you cannot help getting more than you need. Any that you add at the table can only be poisonously excessive.

There is not only experimental but much clinical evidence for the wisdom of this step. Dr. Demetrio Sodi-Pallares of the Institute of Cardiology of Mexico has been using what he calls a "polarizing" therapy much more effective than digitalis compounds, diuretic drugs, and vasodilator agents.

How do you get yourself and your family to adjust to eating without a salt shaker? A mother we know who, out of concern for her family's well being, has made it her business to be nutritionally "on the ball," has succeeded in educating her family away from the salt shaker by promoting "do-it-yourself" seasoning with herbs. She has replaced condiments with attrac-

[351]

tive little containers of oregano, basil, thyme, caraway, sesame, and poppy seeds and invites her family to go creative. Not only are they enjoying their meals more, she says they never seem to miss the salt shaker.

At the same time that we reduce our intake of sodium, it is important that we increase consumption of potassium. Potassium is vital to the life of the cell while sodium is an intruder from the surrounding fluid. When we understand the relationship between the two, we can better enforce a vigorous application of the health rule—low salt, high potassium. When potassium is low, it is as if there were a chink in the cell wall and sodium, always lurking at the gates in the extra-cellular fluid, barges in. The sodium changes the acid-alkaline balance of the cell, making for a toxic condition which fosters the formation of necrotic tissue.

How do you know if you are potassium deficient? Electrocardiographic findings may not be present when the loss is moderate. Even a normal EKG does not exclude the possibility of potassium depletion within the cell. Some of the early symptoms are weakness and impairment of neuromuscular function, absent reflexes, mental confusion, muscles that are soft and sagging like half-filled water bottles. The acne condition of the adolescent whose body is proliferating with new cell growth is a clarion call for more potassium. So is the dry skin of the senior citizen.

Since potassium is present in many foods, one would think a deficiency in our "affluent society" would be unlikely. Such is not the case, says Dr. W. A. Krehl (*Nutrition in Clinical Medicine*, August 22, 1966).

"If food habits had always been sound, the event of potassium deficiency and depletion would not have developed as a major medical problem," he says, and he lays the blame squarely on medical practice for not giving proper emphasis to good dietary habits. Restricted diet selection, misuse of food and inappropriate choice of foods are common faults and account for many of the deficiencies in every stratum of our affluent society.

A diet containing liberal quantities of raw fruits and vegetables may provide adequate dietary intake of potassium with limited amounts of sodium—both desirable objectives. But remember that fruits and vegetables are no better than the soil they are grown on— another factor which may be contributing to potassium deficiency and heart disease. "The plant is the great intermediary by which certain elements of the rocks, after their conversion into soil, are assimilated and made available for the vital processes of animal and man," says C. Growne in *Some Relationships of Soil to Plant and Animal Nutrition.*

Mineral losses through continuous cropping show a reduction of potash (the plant's potassium) over a 5-year period to less than a third. This great loss is typical of many plants and soils and according to Dr. Max Gerson (*Normal Agriculture,* September, 1951) indicates why disease is so prevalent, for potassium deficiency opens the door to acute and chronic diseases.

A large percentage of potassium is bound with protein when subjected to the heat of cooking—making it less available—another reason for the widespread inci-

[353]

dence of potassium deficiency in spite of its generous distribution in nature.

Excellent sources of potassium are bran, corn, eggs, fish, legumes, liver, nuts, oatmeal, bone meal, prunes (especially raw), raisins, whole grains, grapes, yeast, onions, tomatoes, strawberries and especially seeds, seeds, seeds.

You can, as a matter of fact, play a nutritional doubleheader by simply instituting some smart reforms in your snack habits. You can reduce your salt by throwing the potato chips and pretzels to the birds (we wonder if this would be doing our feathered friends a disservice) and fill your snack dishes with seeds— pumpkin, sunflower and sesame, and munch to your heart's content. You will, by this simple substitution, be taking a giant step towards promoting untroubled hearts because all seeds are naturally rich in potassium.

By taking these two steps, reducing salt and increasing potassium, we would, then, according to the evidence, be extending our lease on life. As the late Dr. Tom Douglas Spies said—"If we can help the tissues repair themselves by correcting nutritional deficiencies, we can make old age wait." And, we might add— enjoy that old age without the debilitating handicap of a coronary condition.

[354]

CHAPTER XL

Fish for a Healthier Heart

You can improve your general health and more particularly your heart health, by simply replacing other
protein foods with fish a few times a week. Physicians
at the University of California recently conducted
studies which involved close to 400 men who were
placed on a diet which included 3 to 5 seafood meals
a week over a period of 2 to 3 years. The results were
lowered cholesterol counts, a loss of excess weight and
a general feeling of well-being. The American Heart
Association, in the new booklet, "Reduce Your Risk of
Heart Attack," suggests that a high seafood diet would
be good for anybody.

The relationship between fish and a healthy heart
is not surprising to a nutritionist. Few foods have more
of what it takes to maintain a healthy circulatory system
than seafood. Fish is low in calories; it has almost no

[355]

weight-producing carbohydrates or saturated fats. Its rich supply of unsaturated oils actually helps dissolve any cholesterol accumulations in the blood stream. Fish protein is the best there is, and because protein foods are metabolized more slowly than starchy ones, it satisfies the appetites of overeaters without the accompanying dangers of too much food. Fresh, untreated fish is practically free of sodium, a common restriction for heart patients. If doctors were commissioned to invent the ideal food for a heart patient, chances are they would come up with fish, or something close to it.

Fish is an inexpensive protein source. The protein in any fish is at least as good as meat, but fish is usually cheaper. Fish protein is complete; that is, it supplies all the different kinds of protein elements (amino acids) we need for good health. Compare the amino acids of chicken and beef with fish and you will find that fish has as much or more to offer than either of them.

When you get your protein from fish, 97 per cent of it will be absorbed by your system, and that is 10 per cent more than your system uses from any other source but egg. This wealth of protein works to manufacture hormones and enzymes right in your system, and some of these come ready-made in the fish.

Healthy circulation needs phosphorus—and fish are loaded with it. Without sufficient phosphorus, your body's handling of fat becomes faulty, and so does its ability to metabolize protein. The improper use of fats is, of course, the reason for cholesterol clumps in the

[356]

blood stream, and for eventual hypertension. The necessary amount of phosphorus is essential if the body's supply of calcium is to be used. The calcium is required for proper heart muscle function.

Fish is high in iron, iron that is rapidly absorbed. To the heart patient, iron means more efficient blood composition, and this in turn means less work for the heart. The thyroid gland needs iodine (and fish has plenty) to produce the thyroxine that works toward proper growth, proper use of carbohydrates, quick reactions and normal heart action.

Fish liver oils add to the advantages of seafood for the heart patient. Vitamins A and D are plentiful in these oils, and even the normally scarce vitamin E comes in quantities of 26 to 30 milligrams per 100 grams of oil. The beneficial action of vitamin E is well known for improving the efficiency of the circulatory system, the muscles, and aiding endurance in general. Vitamin A interacts with the essential minerals calcium and phosphorus for improving the heart action and muscle tone. Vitamin A also helps in proper fat storage in the system.

Though the B vitamins have made their reputation as protectors of the nervous system, their effect on the circulation and health of the heart is extremely important. According to the book, *Avitaminosis,* by Walter Eddy, Ph.D. and Gilbert Dalldorf, M.D., "B-vitamin deficiency impairs the function of the heart, increases the tendency to extra-vascular fluid collections and results in terminal cardiac standstill." James S. McLester, M.D., tells of experiments with pigs that

[357]

were fed diets deficient in thiamine (B₁) and showed a scarring of the right side of the heart. (*Nutrition and Diet in Health and Disease,* W. B. Saunders Company)

Beriberi, a disease of vitamin B deficiency, lists heart damage, decreased circulation time, and rise in blood pressure as classic symptoms. The effect of thiamine on the heart and blood vessel system is to increase arterial tone, according to Dr. Walter Eddy. In the face of this information it is comforting to know that the B complex is about as high in fish as in any food, except perhaps the organ meats.

Of course the beneficial action of these nutrients is not tied exclusively to improving or preserving the health of the heart. The proteins, vitamins and minerals of fresh fish offer remarkable dividends in the health of the nerves, bones, skin and other organs. They also protect the body against invading infections and degenerative disorders.

Avoid fresh water fish if at all possible, since these are likely to be infected with the pollution that has increasingly contaminated our inland waterways. As for shellfish (oysters, clams, lobsters, shrimp), *Prevention* considers them a danger in spite of the nutrition they contain. They tend to harbor infectious organisms which are undetectable by the consumer until it is too late.

Americans eat too little fish and perhaps this explains why many of us are actually short of protein. It may explain our high heart disease rate and the vitamin and mineral deficiencies in so many of us. Resolve now

[358]

to change all that for yourself. There are hundreds of different types of fish, and even if you do not enjoy the taste of all fish you can probably find several varieties to your liking. Experiment a bit. Some species are all but free of the fishy smell you might object to and have few hidden bones. Can you think of a cheaper, easier way to insure yourself against heart disease?

CHAPTER XLI

Calcium, Preferably As Bone Meal

It was not until April 14th, 1965 that human knowledge was pushed several steps further along the way to a complete understanding of just how calcium affects the heart and why it is indispensable to that vital organ. On that date Barry Fanburg, M.D., of the Department of Muscle Research of the Retina Foundation in Boston, presented a paper on what he called the "Cardiac Relaxing Factor" to the 48th Annual Meeting of the Federation of American Societies for Experimental Biology. The paper described a study which for the first time has succeeded in determining a good bit about the precise molecular mechanism by which calcium helps the heart to beat and maintains the regularity of that beat.

[360]

Dr. Fanburg's study was based on recent studies from other laboratories that have shown that the contraction of muscles generally depends on two protein elements in the muscle called actin and myosin. These two proteins, acting together, split up a coenzyme, called ATP for short, that is produced in resting muscles. The splitting releases the energy that was formerly involved in bonding the phosphate component to the rest of the compound, and it is this energy that directly activates the muscle.

The process might well be compared to the way energy is released when atoms are split, releasing their binding force. In this case the explosion is a far milder one since it operates on the level of the molecule rather than the atom.

But what has this to do with calcium? That is what Dr. Fanburg set out to discover by extracting actin and myosin from heart muscle and studying under laboratory conditions their ability to cleave ATP.

It was shown that calcium *must be present* in order for actin and myosin to break up ATP and release its bonding energy. And to carry this a step further to its meaning within the human body, the significance of the demonstration was that there must be an ample amount of calcium in the heart in order for the heart to be able to contract with enough force to circulate the blood throughout the body under all conditions.

Does this mean that an insufficient supply of calcium will cause the heart to stop beating? No, it does not. What we have just described is the contraction-producing mechanism in the heart cells that are called

[361]

myofibrils, which are chiefly responsible for energy production. However, the heart is a vital organ and nature has worked out many ways to protect such vital organs. In the case of the heart, nature has endowed it with a secondary mechanism called mitochondria, structures that are able to produce energy by a different mechanism that is not dependent upon calcium. It is this that makes it possible for the heart to go on beating, though perhaps not as efficiently, even when it has been weakened by a lack of calcium. But the basic mechanism in the myofibrils of the heart muscle proper will definitely be weakened by any calcium lack.

We can thus see that calcium plays the role of a kind of catalyst, indispensable for its enzymes to give the heart a strong regular beat. But even more remarkable, Dr. Fanburg has found that it is also calcium that is somehow responsible for the ability of the heart to relax between beats. He has demonstrated that there is in the heart a network of vesicles and tubules which accumulate calcium and which seem to be responsible for the ability of the heart muscle to relax.

Until it becomes possible to study a living, beating heart under a microscope, it will not be possible to describe with certainty the precise mechanism that is involved. In theory, what happens is that the outer network of tubules and vesicles known as "sarcoplasmic reticulum" accumulates calcium and releases it periodically into the muscle fibre. The calcium stimulates contraction of the heart muscle, and when it is used up the muscle relaxes. The heart beats.

What it all goes to show is that the heart—and this

[362]

is equally true of every muscle in the body—requires a good substantial supply of both calcium and phosphorus (needed to form ATP). In order to get them into the body, however, we have to consume them combined in the proper proportions for efficient dietary absorption. And the proper proportions are those that the system itself uses in manufacturing bone. That is why we have long maintained that a regular supplement of bone meal is the best possible way to obtain these vital mineral elements.

There is one other important aspect of Dr. Fanburg's study, though, which also affects the way we fortify ourselves with supplements. He has found that the sarcoplasmic reticulum accumulates not only calcium but also magnesium and there is a presumption in his paper that perhaps the magnesium must be present in order for the calcium to accumulate properly. Whether or not this is so is not known, but we feel it is far better to be safe than cynical. This mineral is of enormous value to heart health. It is quite conceivable and even likely that at least part of this value lies in the affinity between calcium and magnesium and the fact that the sarcoplasmic reticulum must be supplied with both. So to make a real contribution to the health of your heart, we recommend that you also take a dolomite supplement as well as bone meal and make certain that you are getting enough of all three—magnesium, calcium and phosphorus.

[363]

CHAPTER XLII

An Amino-Acid Improves Hearts

One of the most fascinating aspects of the developing new knowledge of amino acids and what can be done with them is the number of important uses that are being found for the so-called non-essential amino acids. The twelve amino acids falling into this category are just as necessary to health and to normal growth, regeneration and reproduction as are the ten "essential" amino acids. The only difference is that our diets must furnish all ten of the essential amino acids to the full extent that health and life require them, while the non-essential ones can be manufactured within our own bodies. Our bodies do not necessarily manufacture enough of them, however, and there is reason to believe that the non-essential amino acids are every bit as important in our everyday diets as the essential.

[364]

A good example is aspartic acid, a non-essential amino acid about which little is known and which doctors generally do not consider of any importance at all. It is one of the food elements that are stripped out of sugar cane, in which it is abundant, in the manufacture of "purified" table sugar. Present in many protein foods, it is abundant only in asparagus among the foods that are readily available to us.

Have you ever had a doctor tell you that you ought to eat more asparagus for better health? Or have you ever heard a doctor complain that sugar refining reduces the amount of aspartic acid available in our diets? Of course not. Doctors have long accepted the idea that the non-essential amino acids are of no importance. It is only now and very slowly that they are learning otherwise.

What are they learning?

One illuminating article on the values of aspartic acid, both for therapy and in normal health, appeared in a book published in Switzerland by S. Karger in 1965. A symposium titled *Electrolytes and Cardiovascular Diseases*, it contains one article by two French doctors, M. Lamarche and R. Royer, that specifically reports on the value of aspartic acid to the heart.

These doctors set out to check on earlier reports that when the coronary arteries of rabbits were tied off, reducing the blood supply to the heart, the consequent fluttering and increase of the heartbeat had been found to be reduced when aspartic acid was introduced into the organism. "We studied the aspartate protection of the guinea pig heart with regard to the myocardial

[365]

mechanical function and the ECG (electrocardiogram) modifications occurring under the influence of
hypoxia (insufficient oxygen) and anoxia (no oxygen)." What Lamarche and Royer found was a "therapeutic cardiac action." They were able to determine,
in other words, that aspartic acid does slow down the
heart in a distress situation and that it does this fundamentally by reducing the need of the heart for oxygen.

The authors go on to describe their experiments:

After devising a technique to make certain that the
heart was receiving a regular but insufficient amount of
oxygen, they confirmed that this situation caused the
heart to beat faster with a shallower beat. Each contraction would thus circulate less blood, which the
heart attempted to compensate for by increasing the
number of contractions. Perfusion of the heart with a
solution containing aspartic acid, however, caused the
amplitude or the amount of power in each beat to
increase, permitting a slowing down of the number of
beats per minute.

Then turning to the actual amount of blood flowing
through the coronary artery and measuring it, it was
found that even with an insufficiency of oxygen, aspartic acid induced the heart to maintain a normal
flow of blood.

These results were obtained, confirmed and recon-
firmed by readings on the electrocardiograph.

In discussing their work, the authors say that their
results "demonstrate by their agreement of unquestion-
able cardiac action of certain aspartic acid salts." What
this action basically consists of is that "the amplitude

[366]

of the cardiac contraction is regularly increased. . . ." And they go on to point out that this means that aspartic acid enables the heart to do more work with less strain. Or as the authors put it, "The aspartates are energy-sparing and improve the cardiac efficiency requiring less energy for more work."

And the authors conclude by pointing out the therapeutic use to which the results of their study can be put. They recommend "Use of this drug in cardiac insufficiency and hyposystolia; by bringing up the improvement of efficiency without increase in the coronary blood flow, by emphasizing the protection of the isolated organ and the whole animal against the effects of hypoxia and acute anoxia immediately one imagines therapeutic change in chronic coronary insufficiency."

The authors also point out that there is a difference between laboratory animals and human beings which may sometimes be significant. They recommend further studies and attempts to treat human coronary insufficiency with aspartic acid. It is to be hoped that the medical profession will follow up their lead.

It has already been found by some of the most important doctors in France (Laborit, Coirault, Thiebault and Vial) that the potassium and magnesium salts of aspartic acid bring about a definite increase in available energy and a corresponding reduction in fatigue. The method by which this is accomplished is still unknown, but the effect is important and its harmlessness has been established.

In efforts to investigate the mechanism of this effect, it has been found that aspartic acid plays a key role

[367]

in one of the important detoxifications that regularly go on in the body. Because our crops are excessively treated with nitrate fertilizers, we all have large amounts of ammonia in our systems, coming from the foods that we eat. Aspartic acid is necessary to transform the ammonia to urea, in which form it is filtered out of the bloodstream by the kidneys and excreted by the urine. If we lack an adequate amount of aspartic acid, we will find it impossible to get rid of all the ammonia in our systems and it may well be the accumulation of ammonia that is one of the causes of chronic fatigue. It is a wonderful reason for eating more asparagus.

Can this same ability to detoxify ammonia be responsible for the beneficent effect aspartic acid has on the heart? It would be very hard to say at this point. There just have not been enough studies made.

Even with the little that has been discovered so far, however, it has already become apparent that aspartic acid is destined to play an important role in the medical treatments of the future.

Eat more asparagus.

CHAPTER XLIII

The Power of Pectin

Rutgers University's Department of Nutrition recently announced that pectin, a carbohydrate found in the cell walls of many fruits and vegetables, may be an important factor in the prevention of heart disease. Drs. Hans Fisher and Paul Griminger, quoted in the *Farm Journal* (April, 1968), state that pectin limits the amount of cholesterol the body can absorb, and thus tends to limit that dangerous accumulation of cholesterol in the bloodstream. The high pectin count in apples, suggests the *Journal,* may be one of the reasons for its reputed ability to keep the doctor away.

The power of pectin is not news to *Prevention* readers. In September, 1961, we reported the findings of Dr. Ancel Keys of the University of Minnesota that ". . . Controlled experiments on man have shown that pectin in the diet has a small but definite effect on lowering blood cholesterol levels. In these experiments

[369]

carried out on four groups of middle-aged men in a state hospital, the addition to the daily diet of 15 grams (about half an ounce) of pure pectin caused the blood cholesterol to fall by an average of about 5 per cent. When the pectin was removed from this diet the blood cholesterol promptly rose to the prepectin level." Dr. Keys remarked that pectin is naturally contained in many fruits and berries, notably apples. He said that the amount of pectin used in these experiments would be provided by about two pounds of apples. "It appears probable, however, that the high consumption of fruits, including apples, by some populations, helps to explain the low blood cholesterol values in these populations . . ."

Studies on animals have also shown that pectin added to the diet apparently will reduce the absorption of cholesterol from the intestines, therefore allowing the cholesterol to pass through the body and be excreted. In another group of experiments the scientists found that animals fed cholesterol one day and pectin the next responded with a lowering of the serum cholesterol as compared with animals fed no pectin. It appeared from the findings of these doctors that the pectin encouraged and increased elimination of the cholesterol in fecal matter.

Edna Brown Southmayd, Ph.D., reported some years ago (*Nutrition Research,* December, 1961) on just how pectin does its job. "As the plant matures, enzyme action within the plant releases soluble and consequently digestible pectin substances. Pectin has a strong water-binding property, which helps plants to retain their

[370]

water and makes it useful in making jellies. Interestingly, it is the pectin of green fruit, which is indigestible, that has this jellying property. The pectin of more mature fruit, which we do digest, for that very reason of its solubility, is not good for jelly making. This is probably one of the important factors entering into the established fact that ripe fruits and vegetables are more fully digested than green ones."

Russian researchers say the pectin derived from sunflowers is superior, according to the USSR publication, *Labor Hygiene and Occupational Diseases.* The Russians did not state whether the pectin used in their experiments was from mature or unripe sunflower seeds. However, we have long believed that, in addition to their known superb nutritional value, there are in sunflower seeds many as yet undiscovered or unconfirmed properties.

There is also evidence that pectin is a detoxifier: "It has been known for more than a hundred years that the ingestion of pectin would prevent lead poisoning. This, according to Dr. Glenn H. Joseph (*Nutrition Research,* September, 1955), is because pectin, in the digestive process, is transformed into galacturonic acid, which has the property of combining with certain heavy metals into insoluble metallic salts. These salts cannot be absorbed into the system and so they are excreted. Galacturonic acid from pectin combines in the same way with calcium, causing its excretion and, since we know that calcium and strontium 90 are molecular twins, we might speculate even without any evidence that pectin might be expected to combine, as galactu-

[371]

ronic acid, with strontium 90 and prevent it from being absorbed into the system. . . . There is no need to wait for proof so far as our diets are concerned. The consumption of foods containing pectin will not do any harm and strong nutritional benefits make it important in every diet."

Dr. Edwin F. Bryant, Ph.D. explains that pectin removes toxic wastes from the body by combining with them into chemical forms that permit their elimination. It also clears constipation, says Bryant, by its water binding properties, moistening and softening the wastes to be eliminated.

Pectin nourishes the intestinal flora, helping it to carry on the vital work of combating and controlling the number of disease bacteria. The pectin, in its turn, is converted by these benign bacteria into fatty acids which arrest the development of the bacteria responsible for bacillary dysentery, infantile diarrhea and other intestinal disorders. Some of the pectin entering the intestines combines with calcium to form calcium gels, which aid healthy elimination by providing bulk.

In 1965 Italy produced an interesting applesauce-anti-cholesterol experiment. Three Italian doctors of Santa Anna Main Hospital, Ferrara, Italy turned the coincidence of a plentiful apple crop and a comparatively high cholesterol level in the area of their hospital to advantage. Within two to three weeks these apples alone brought about a reduction in cholesterol in 32 experimental patients.

Research began by investigating changes in the cholesterol levels of chickens when a certain amount of grated apple was added to their cholesterol-rich diet. The chickens responded so well that it was decided to take the apple approach with humans. Two to three apples after each meal were added to the diets of 26 in-patients and 6 out-patients at Santa Anna Main Hospital. It worked out to about 200 grams (7 ounces) of blended or grated apple pulp. Only a few of the patients actually munched whole apples.

To make certain that it was the apples alone, the full diet was continued unchanged in every other respect, including some high cholesterol foods. Tests made at the beginning and at the end cf the dietetic course showed that cholesterol levels that went down with apples went up in some patients several days after the apple treatment was discontinued.

Doctors noted that the way the apples were prepared —blended, grated, or cut into chewable slices—influenced the amount of serum cholesterol differently. The finer the pulp the greater the surface of apple quickly exposed to the intestines, and the plainer were the results in blood cholesterol reduction.

The Italians were unanimous in their opinion that the pectin content of apples is the element responsible for stabilizing the cholesterol levels.

Housewives know that pectin is what it takes to make the jelly gel. In the days when pectin wasn't available commercially, cooks used to combine apples with whatever fruit they were using for jelly and jams. There was always enough pectin in the apples to get the fruit and sugar mix to gel. Of course the amount of pectin one gets in the average serving of jelly or jam is inconse-

[373]

quential, so don't count on it to have an effect on dangerous cholesterol levels.

To put these discoveries of the value of pectin to good use, eat apples. Eat lots of apples. Eat them raw and unprocessed. We think you should peel them because, unless they are organically grown, they have been heavily sprayed. . . . If, because of some condition of health, you aren't able to chew raw apples, liquefy them in a blender just before eating them. If you have no blender, scrape the cored peeled apple with a dull knife and eat the scrapings. You will find that raw apples are wonderfully satisfying to eat—so satisfying that you won't want to eat the pastries and other desserts that contain the overload of fat which everybody, including Dr. Ancel Keys, believes is so destructive to health. Other fresh, raw fruits and berries contain pectin, but apples are the richest source.

CHAPTER XLIV

Soybeans and Eggs for Lecithin

Ever since medicine became cholesterol-conscious, doctors have been experimenting with methods of bringing high levels within the normal bounds—between 200 to 300 milligrams per 100 cubic centimeters of blood for most Americans. Some physicians tell their patients to cut out foods that are high in cholesterol. This includes eggs, fish roe, kidney, liver, sweetbreads and others—the very foods rich in vitamins and minerals we all need desperately. Others have tried to lower cholesterol with drugs that sometimes caused disastrous consequences.

A far better approach, it seems to us, would be to study the patient's whole diet to see if he is getting too little of some essential element his body needs to metabolize cholesterol properly. Lecithin is such a factor, and soybeans are one food that has plenty of it.

A soybean compound was fed to prison volunteers

[375]

and students in a recent dietary experiment conducted by Dr. Robert E. Hodges, Professor of Medicine at the University of Iowa, Iowa City. Dr. Hodges reported that the blood cholesterol level of the subjects dropped from an average of about 300 milligrams per cent to 200 or less. He told the convention of the American Societies of Experimental Biology, April 13, 1966, that the tests had proven diet alone, aside from greater physical activity, could lead to lower blood cholesterol levels.

A prominent Los Angeles internist, Lester M. Morrison, M.D., has published his conviction that lecithin not only reduces the amount of cholesterol in the blood, but actually reverses the process known as atherosclerosis—the building up of fatty deposits in the vital arteries of the heart and head. Dr. Morrison stated, "It has been demonstrated that lecithin can lower the lipid (fat) levels of the blood, but there seems to be good evidence now that in very high concentrations lecithin can also dissolve the fatty plaques in the arteries."

In his book, *The Low-Fat Way to Health and Longer Life,* Morrison points out that until recently it was believed that once fatty deposits imbedded themselves in the artery walls, things could only get worse. As the passageway narrowed, a clot could form on the roughened surface of the arteries' inner lining and could stop the flow of blood altogether, resulting in a coronary attack or a stroke. Now experiments with lecithin have proven that this is not necessarily so.

It is interesting that egg yolk is rich in cholesterol as well as in lecithin. Could it be that nature attempts to

[376]

insure cholesterol's proper use by coupling it with lecithin so that the body can handle it with ease? Perhaps the cholesterol problem would never have come up if it were not for the way we process our food. Hydrogenated fats, for example, are loaded with cholesterol, but the hydrogenation process all but eliminates the lecithin they originally contained.

Lecithin acts as an emulsifying agent for cholesterol. When cholesterol tends to coalesce or lump together, the lecithin breaks it up, mixes with it and keeps it divided into tiny particles so that it can circulate through the body without solidifying or congealing into larger particles. Without lecithin there is nothing to keep cholesterol from caking or lumping and clinging to the sides of the arteries.

Early in the heart disease-cholesterol debate, the *American Journal of Digestive Diseases* (April, 1952) published the work of Pottenger and Krohn who went against the common trend of low-fat diets to cut high cholesterol. They gave their patients the opposite, a diet high in fat and cholesterol—plus lecithin from soybeans. Out of 122 patients put on a high fat diet that included raw liver and raw brains—foods high in cholesterol—99 of the patients took a teaspoon of soybean lecithin with each meal. The remaining 23, serving as controls, did not take the soybean preparation.

"The blood cholesterol showed a marked decrease in 79 per cent of patients who took the lecithin, but not in the patients who did not take lecithin."

Many people who suspect that they consume too much in the way of hydrogenated fats, and have a cho-

[377]

lesterol reading that is higher than it should be, include lecithin in their diets as a food supplement. Lecithin, used in this way, is made chiefly from soybeans. In fact, soya-lecithin has come to be the name generally used for lecithin because it is practically always made from soybeans.

Soybeans themselves are a wonderfully nutritious food. For some reason, Americans neglect them in spite of the rich protein they contain and their important vitamin content. Soybeans offer large amounts of calcium, iron and other trace minerals as well as precious B vitamins and vitamin E. Particularly plentiful: two of the B vitamins, choline and pantothenic acid, and the vital lecithin.

The fresh green soybeans are cooked much as any other fresh beans are cooked. Dried soybeans, which can be stored the way Navy beans are, require a soaking period, and are prepared just the way other beans are prepared. Soybeans are not starchy. They may be used as a vegetable, or, because of their high protein content, they may occasionally be served in place of meat or eggs. Your family should become familiar with this interesting and healthful food as soon as possible.

[378]

CHAPTER XLV

Raw Fruits and Vegetables

In all the flurry over whether fats in the diet are responsible for heart trouble and hardening of the arteries, all the debates raging as to whether this fat or that is responsible for the thickened walls of arteries, while one side cries out "animal fats are responsible" and the other insists that diets high in fat of any kind are the guilty parties it is refreshing to come upon an entirely new theory about heart disease and hardening of the arteries, developed by W. J. McCormick, M.D. and published in the July, 1957 issue of *Clinical Medicine.*

Dr. McCormick has what you might call an obsession with the subject of vitamin C. And who can blame him? He has devoted so much study to this subject, has done so many tests on the average level of vitamin C in his patients and has achieved such remarkable results in treating patients with this elusive and mysterious substance that we feel we can always look to him for something new and stimulating on the subject. The article referred to is no exception.

Coronary thrombosis, one of the most prevalent causes of death in our age, is defined as a clotting of blood in the artery that runs to the heart, caused usually by a slowing of the circulation or changes in the blood or blood-vessel walls. If the blood cannot pass this clot, the patient may die, since the heart needs fresh blood every moment. What causes the blood to clot? There are different opinions on this, says Dr. McCormick. He quotes E. Ziegler in a book *General Pathology* as saying that when the inner wall of the blood vessel is injured by compression, crushing or irritant chemicals, certain parts of the blood attach themselves to the wall at that point and assist in the healing process so that eventually the point of damage looks like just a healthy thickening in the wall. However, under present circumstances, Dr. McCormick goes on, the injured place fails to heal properly and the material that collects may form into a clot that closes off the blood vessel entirely.

In much of the scientific investigation of hardening of the arteries, researchers have found that a disturbance in the actual substance of the artery wall is common to all. The wall is weakened, becomes fragile and may rupture, resulting in hemorrhages. A similar condition is characteristic of vitamin C deficiency.

J. C. Paterson reported in the *Canadian Medical Association Journal,* volume 44, page 114, 1941, that 81 per cent of coronary patients in a hospital studied

[380]

had a subnormal level of vitamin C in their blood as compared to only 55.8 per cent of a corresponding group with assorted diseases. Other investigators have found that various conditions involving stress have resulted in blood clots forming. We know that stress creates greater demand for vitamin C. Tests have showed that people and animals with scurvy (the disease of vitamin C deficiency) have deposits of cholesterol in their blood vessels like those present in hardening of the arteries. One investigator, indeed, found widespread hardening of the arteries and blood clots in young people in prison camps where the diet was certainly not high in cholesterol, but must have been low in vitamin C. So it seems that lack of vitamin C must play an important part in the whole story.

When vitamin C is deficient, the intercellular cement substance becomes semi-liquid and a protein it contains is released into the blood stream. This protein is found in the blood stream during a wide variety of disorders—the rheumatic diseases, shock, burns, physical injuries, infections, cancer and certain heart conditions. It is also true that a deficiency of vitamin C is found in patients with these conditions and that patients who have them have a tendency to blood clots.

J. B. Duguid, writing in *The Lancet,* page 6818, 1954, is quoted by Dr. McCormick as saying that the incidence of coronary disease did not decline in Great Britain during the war when the intake of fat was restricted, nor, for that matter, can one produce hardening of the arteries by feeding animals the amount of cholesterol that might be found in a diet high in fat.

[381]

J. B. Wolffe, in the *New York State Journal of Medicine,* volume 56, page 2361, 1956, said, "A high fat and high cholesterol intake is no more the cause of atherosclerosis than a high carbohydrate intake is the cause of diabetes mellitus."

If indeed vitamin C deficiency may be responsible for hardening of the arteries, how is it possible that all or even any of those hundreds of thousands dying of coronary thrombosis today could be possibly short in vitamin C? This is the question that comes immediately to mind. Isn't it true that we have practically eliminated scurvy as such?

We have seen that "stress" depletes the body of vitamin C. Anything poisonous to the human body increases its production of a substance manufactured by the adrenal glands, which uses up vitamin C. Exposure to the stress of surgery may thus be responsible for blood clots after operations. Poisons like certain chemicals and nicotine act the same way.

On the subject of nicotine, Dr. McCormick has some very interesting statistics. In a study of 151 fatal cases of coronary thrombosis 97 per cent had been smokers; 58 per cent had been heavy smokers. Their average age at death was 47. The 42 per cent who had been light or moderate smokers had an average age at death of 58½ years. In a recent American Cancer Society survey it was found that the number of deaths from coronary thrombosis was almost twice as high in the cigarette smokers as in the non-smokers. Buerger's Disease, a disorder of the blood vessels which, if not controlled, may necessitate amputation of affected limbs, is almost entirely a disease of smokers and, in many cases, the cessation of smoking alone has stopped the disease in its tracks. Buerger's Disease used to be a man's disease —extremely uncommon in women. Recently there has been a leveling off and women are more and more susceptible to the disease. Of course women are also smoking more with every passing year.

The same general trend in statistics prevails where coronary thrombosis is concerned. Prior to 1929 the sex ratio of incidence was estimated at about 7 males to 1 female. Recent figures from the Toronto Health Department indicate this ratio to be only 2 to 1 at present. More women are smoking; more women are dying of coronary thrombosis. Dr. McCormick does not say that smoking alone is the cause of this change. But he does point out that cigarette consumption was 5 billion in 1935 and 25 billion in 1955, an increase of 500 per cent. In this same time the population increased 40 per cent. The same has been true in the United States. There has been no such increase in the consumption of cholesterol-rich foods during this period, Dr. McCormick points out.

He reminds us again that in careful records kept over his long life in medicine he has found that about 90 per cent of his patients are deficient in vitamin C. He reminds us again of laboratory tests showing that the smoking of one cigarette destroys in the body about as much vitamin C as you obtain from the average orange.

What is the lesson to be learned from Dr. McCormick's startling and provocative theory? Should readers

[383]

immediately rush out and buy an electric fryer and start eating hydrogenated fats and French fries at every meal, safe in the conviction that the wrong kind of fats cannot possibly harm one's heart and circulatory system? Certainly not. We are sure nothing could be further from the intent of Dr. McCormick's article.

Instead, let us contemplate soberly some further facts along these lines. Isn't it true that folks who eat lots of pies, pastry, fried foods, desserts and other things rich in the wrong kind of fats are those most likely to be short on vitamin C? There isn't any vitamin C in such foods, you know, and everyone has a certain capacity. As you gradually drop such foods from your menus you will find automatically that you are eating more fresh fruits, more salads, more raw vegetables. And this will give you more vitamin C.

If you feel that you are already getting plenty of vitamin C in your daily meals so you don't have to worry about the possibility of deficiency, sit down and study carefully all the various substances to which you are exposed every day which may be using up your vitamin C faster than you are supplying it to your body.

Do you travel in automobiles, breathing carbon monoxide gas? Ever sit in a room where someone is smoking? Are you exposed to such things as paint fumes, benzene products, insecticides, drugs of any kind? Do you get your fruits and vegetables fresh from your garden and eat them raw with only the briefest washings? Or do you, like most of us, have to buy fruits and vegetables at the store where they may have been resting for weeks while their vitamin C content evaporates?

[384]

There is no way you can possibly know just what is the exact vitamin content of the food you have bought, you know, in spite of all the tables giving average vitamin content. And of course practically all food contains insecticides.

Now add to this the certain fact that each of us is subject to stress—even cold or hot weather, fatigue, worry, fright—these are stress conditions. They create a greater demand for vitamin C in your body.

So the lesson to be learned from Dr. McCormick's thinking on heart disease and vitamin C is to keep your diet as healthful as possible—high in protein, low in fats, especially animal fats and processed fats, and high in fresh raw fruits and vegetables. If you really eat a diet like this you needn't worry for you are omitting the fats which may be dangerous and you are getting quantities of the vitamin which may protect against disorders of the blood vessels and heart—vitamin C.

In addition, just because you can't be absolutely sure how much vitamin C you are getting, especially in winter, do take a natural vitamin C supplement, made from rose hips, green peppers or some other rich source.

[385]

CHAPTER XLVI

Quit Drinking Coffee

J. I. Rodale

The heart cannot stand alone. It is part of the whole body. If something is wrong in the rest of the system, the task of the heart is more arduous. It is working up-hill, against odds. If there is high blood pressure, for example, or diabetes, or kidney trouble, or something that is raising the pulse, then every beat the heart takes is done with greater effort. It is important, therefore, that a heart case give up coffee drinking, so as to insure that no other pathological conditions will arise to impose an additional burden on the heart. But coffee drinking is bad for the heart itself, as you shall see.

Of all the harm that coffee drinking does, its ability to prevent iron from being utilized in the body, is one of the more serious disadvantages. A doctor writing to *The Lancet* (December 7, 1957) says, "It is indeed

[386]

rather difficult to understand how people who take tea or coffee with every meal can ever absorb iron from their food at all." This could lead to anemia which is a rather unpleasant complication for a heart case.

Then there is the question of a possible vitamin deficiency caused by coffee drinking. Walter H. Eddy, Ph.D. in his book *Vitaminology* (Williams and Wilkins) says it may be that large amounts of caffeine in coffee may create an inositol deficiency. Inositol is one of the B complex vitamins. The coffee bean contains from 1 to 2 per cent caffeine. It has been reported, says Dr. Eddy, that when commercial coffee was added to the basal diet of dogs, a paralysis resulted that was curable by inositol. An eye condition also occurred that could be corrected by giving biotin, another of the B vitamins. The suggestion is that the inclusion of caffeine in the diet can create a biotin and inositol deficiency.

A confirmation of this fact is in an article in *Archives of Bio-chemistry*, 1945, vol. 6, entitled "Studies on the Nicotinic Acid Content of Coffee," which proves that drinking coffee could produce a vitamin deficiency.

Drugs and certain soluble chemicals have been known to use up some of the body's vitamin resources. Chlorine uses up vitamin E, alcohol vitamin B, tobacco vitamin C. Now we see that caffeine has a similar power, and for that reason it is absolutely contra-indicated to a heart case, for such deficiencies can cause serious disorders in the body that may make it more difficult for the heart to function efficiently.

Caffeine as a drug is used by the medical profession in certain cases of heart trouble. It dilates the coronary

[387]

arteries, and furnishes a better blood supply to the heart. Many heart cases will experience a sense of comfort with coffee, but this is the short-term effect. What is its effect on the long pull?

In this respect I would like to relate my own experience. For a long time I came to lean rather heavily on coffee, drinking 8 cups a day, and it worked wonderfully as far as my heart condition was concerned. When I gave it up on several occasions I would begin to experience chest angina pains on exertion. But when I went back to coffee this condition would miraculously clear up. Of course basically it was the vitamin E that I was taking that prevented these symptoms, but coffee was doing its share too. One seemed to be no good without the other. So I went about singing the praises of coffee, and feeling that perhaps it was saving my life.

But something was happening to me that made me question the use of coffee. In the first place I was becoming very nervous. Secondly, I seemed to be experiencing difficulty in remembering things. I would meet a person on the street whom I knew rather intimately and for the life of me, I wouldn't be able to think of his name. Caffeine, I knew, destroys nerve cells and I could see that it was beginning to do a rather good job on mine, especially the ones in my brain.

Now I began to realize that drinking coffee could be a powerful contributor to the senility of old age, the doddering of the mind and the body in general. Dr. Frederick C. Swartz, of Lansing, Michigan, in a discussion of physical health at the University of Michigan recently said that if a person wished to avoid shaky

[388]

hands and a tottering gait in later life he should give up drinking coffee.

As far as my heart was concerned, coffee drinking didn't seem to hurt it. On the contrary it seemed to help. It didn't raise my pulse even one beat a minute. But I feared some hidden damage that it could be doing which would make my heart suffer later in the period near the last lap when my heart would want every organ of my body to play ball properly.

I decided to cut out drinking coffee for the third time, and did it in November, 1956. I watched for the return of my heart symptoms as had occurred twice before, that time I did not experience them. Evidently my program of healthy living, daily exercise, walking an hour a day, taking my vitamins and following a generally healthy nutritional program had strengthened my heart, so that this time it didn't require coffee as a prop. And slowly my nervousness began to disappear and my ability to remember improve. As the months go by, I feel better and better, but it will take many years to do away completely with the damage that coffee did to my body.

One of the most dangerous drawbacks of coffee drinking is the false sense of security it gives to a heart case. You drink a cup of coffee and you feel as if you're sailing on the clouds. Actually your physical body is still tired, the way it was before you drank your coffee. Therefore, instead of sitting down you are up and about. That is what killed my oldest brother Archie who died at 51 of a heart attack. He had just finished lunch, topped off with the usual cups of coffee, and

[389]

felt so full of energy that he began to repair a chair. He keeled over in a heart attack and was dead in minutes.

Coffee drinking is like using a whip on a tired horse. Of course he will move faster but how long will he go before he drops from exhaustion? The heart case is whipping himself with cups of coffee but eventually the ledger account must be adjusted.

Max M. Rosenberg, M.D. in *The Encyclopedia of Medical Self Help* tells us that coffee should be avoided by individuals who have heart trouble, angina, high blood pressure, stomach trouble, skin affections, arthritis and liver trouble.

According to James S. McLester, M.D. in his book *Nutrition and Diet in Health and Disease* (W. B. Saunders, 1927) excessive use of coffee is harmful. He says that in cases of cardiac irritability and rapid heart beat, even one cup a day will cause trouble, for the heart is already irritated.

H. M. Marvin, M.D., in his book *You and Your Heart* (Random House, 1950) states that the effect of coffee varies among different individuals. Some find that their heart beats faster, but others do not. Some people seem to develop a tolerance for coffee, but there are hidden effects that may not appear on the surface. One can "get away with" coffee drinking up to a certain age perhaps, but what is the cumulative effect of the caffeine at later ages, and exactly what is the danger point as far as age is concerned?

Horst, Burton and Robinson, in The *Journal of Pharmacology and Experimental Therapeutics*, vol. 52, 1934 tell of an experience involving a number of young men whose blood pressure was tested before and after they began to drink coffee habitually. The maximum rise in blood pressure occurred during the first week they were drinking coffee. Later on, a tolerance was developed, and the blood pressure remained at the same level. When the coffee was withdrawn, the blood pressure returned to normal. This experiment shows that in many persons some substance in coffee does have an unhealthful effect on the blood pressure.

Dr. Jean Bogert in her textbook *Nutrition and Physical Fitness* (W. B. Saunders, 1949) says that coffee drinking raises the blood pressure. Garfield G. Duncan, M.D., in *Diseases of Metabolism* (W. B. Saunders, 1952) says that caffeine causes an increase of 3 to 10 per cent in the basal metabolic rate of the body within the first hour after the coffee is taken. (So, incidentally, does the smoking of one cigarette.) This means that the processes of the body have been quickened to that extent. But is that desirable where there is a heart condition?

A heart case should be very careful how he cuts out coffee drinking, if he has come to depend on it. If he experiences any symptoms, then he must go on a rigorous program of developing his body the way I did. Temporarily he might have to reduce the number of cups a day, or drink half cups. But gradually, through careful body conditioning, he is bound to conquer the habit without distressing his heart.

Tea is just as bad as coffee, but there are many other hot drinks available such as postum, mint, carob, and herbal teas. My favorite is rose hip tea.

[391]

CHAPTER XLVII

Put Away the Salt Shaker

Some people make more use of a salt shaker when they eat than they do of a knife and fork. The plate has hardly set to rest on the table before they pass the salt shaker over everything on it. They put salt on watermelon and cantaloupe; ham and fish, often naturally too salty, get the full treatment anyway. Only the coffee escapes, and oftentimes the cook has taken care of that by adding salt to the grounds before brewing, to "enhance" the flavor. For such people what lies under the salt is incidental. It could be a rubber sponge as well as a hamburger, or soap suds as well as mashed potatoes. If the consistency is similar, the taste will be the same—salty.

Of course these people are missing a large part of the pleasure of eating—the subtle flavor of fresh foods, not masked by any condiments. If that were all they are missing, it would not be the concern of the nutritionist.

[392]

Much more is involved, however. The addition of salt to foods is a health hazard so serious that death can result from its overuse.

While it is true that no death certificate ever gave "salt" as cause of death, heart failure, hypertension, enlarged heart and kidney failure appear quite often, and anyone of these can be the result of high salt intake. A quite convincing illustration of the dangers salt holds appeared in the *Annals of Internal Medicine* (November, 1953). In this article four doctors reported on their findings in an experiment to determine the effect of various salt rations—on a selected group of healthy rats. Seven groups were included in the test. The first group was fed a diet which contained about twice as much salt as the minimum considered absolutely necessary to sustain life. A second group ate a diet with the usual amount of salt used in all nutritional experiments. The amount was increased with each of the other five groups—20, 40, 50, 60 and 70 times the amount needed to sustain life.

After two months, 18 per cent of the rats in the three groups highest in salt intake had shown edema (unhealthy swelling) and an abrupt increase in weight. When these rats were sacrificed for further study, their kidneys were seen damaged in much the same fashion as in human cases of nephritis. The blood pressure of these rats had shown an increase and profound anemia was evident; blood protein was low.

The experiment continued. At the end of nine months hypertensive animals appeared in all of the five groups who had salt in their diets which exceeded

[393]

the usual amount in laboratory diets. Most animals in the groups with the highest increases of salt had striking rises in blood pressure. It was obvious that the relationship between salt increase and blood pressure increase was proportionate. Chronic kidney failure was also common among the higher salt intake groups.

Of course these experiments were carried on with rats, not people, and some will deny that the results apply to humans. But it must be admitted that salt does cause all tissue to hold water and increase body weight. Weight is a major factor in human heart disease because of the extra work it imposes on the heart. Excess sodium does create hardships for the kidneys. These facts hold good for men as well as rats, and we only show good sense when we heed the warnings presented by such experiments.

Without salt the body's functioning would soon stop completely. We need a certain amount of it. But this amount is really quite small—2 to 3 grams per day, according to R. Ackerly, M.D., in the *Proceedings of the Royal Society of Medicine,* 1910. We eat an average of 7 to 10 times that much and often more. Dr. L. Duncan Bulkley, editor of the journal *Cancer,* believes that one can do very well on 7 grams of added salt per week. These 7 grams come to one easily, without so much as touching the salt shaker. Just the sodium that is added to today's foods in processing would well fill the average family's needs. Add to this the salt used in the kitchen as the cook puts a meal together, and the 7 grams per week has been met and surpassed.

In the June 5, 1959 issue of the *New England Jour-*

nal of Medicine, Lewis K. Dahl, M.D. gave some interesting information on salt and salt intake. He says that while high blood pressure can be induced in animals by injecting certain chemicals, these chemicals will cause high blood pressure only if salt makes up 2-4 per cent of the daily diet. Dr. Dahl along with Robert A. Love, M.D., also published a paper in the *Journal of the American Medical Association* (May 25, 1957), showing high blood pressure to be much more frequent among those humans who eat lots of salt as compared to those who are on low salt diets. They made careful observations on a total of 1,346 adults before writing this article. They divided the individuals (all employees of the laboratory) into three groups: those who denied ever adding salt to food at the table; those who added salt if, after tasting it, they found it "needed" salt; and those who automatically added salt to everything they ate without tasting it first. They called these groups "low," "average" and "high" in their consumption of salt—which seems to us a very fair way of naming them.

"Hypertension" was defined as blood pressure of at least 140/90. And of course, all figures over that level. The results of the observations (kept over a period of years) showed some very significant facts about salt-eating and high blood pressure. The authors found, first of all, that individuals who are not overweight but are on a high-salt diet will have several times the incidence of hypertension, or high blood pressure, found in similar persons on a low-salt diet. 2. Among individuals who are on a high-salt diet, those who are overweight will

[395]

have considerably more high blood pressure than those who are not overweight. 3. Those people who are both overweight and on a high-salt diet will have a much greater incidence of hypertension than will those not overweight and on a low-salt diet.

It is known, say the authors, that overweight individuals suffer from hypertension more commonly than do people of normal weight. Could it be, they ask, that in eating more food generally, more salt is taken? They feel this is one possible explanation.

In no case was there any real craving for salt in patients whose intake was drastically reduced. For a week or so they complained that food tasted flat, but after that they became used to the new flavors and there were no more complaints. For some the experience of giving up salt is similar to that of giving up smoking and drinking. For the first week or so the memory of old tastes persists, and after that one simply forgets that they existed and has no desire for their return.

The high blood pressures indicated in the rats on salt diets, quoted above, have a counterpart in 21 patients reported on in *Ugeskrift For Laeger,* a Copenhagen journal for March 30, 1950. These were treated with a low salt diet for 1 to 5 months. In all cases blood pressure was reduced 20 to 75 mm., usually within 2 to 4 weeks.

One of the current arguments against salt intake is offered by Dr. Abraham E. Nizel in his book, *Nutrition and Clinical Dentistry.* He asserts that excess sodium chloride (salt) will enter into a struggle with calcium

[396]

in the body and win. The result is less than an adequate amount of calcium for healthy teeth and bones. In this roundabout way we have excessive use of salt to thank for dental caries. And calcium is also essential to heart health.

Among other interesting effects of salt intake, we saw the strong guess by Dr. Eugene Foldes, printed in the *Medical Journal of Australia* (May 31, 1958), that baldness is one. Dr. Foldes did an experiment in which, in a closed environment, he actually counted the hairs falling from a subject eating salt without restriction. When the salt intake was reduced, the hairs falling out decreased in number. However, upon resumption of the unrestricted salt intake the number of falling hairs increased in 2 days. Are you balding? Do you eat a lot of added salt?

Insomnia is also related to salt intake, in the opinion of a French Army doctor, Professor Coirault. In a speech before a conference on mental hygiene, he told of this theory based on the fact that sodium and potassium are natural enemies in the body's chemistry. He said that a cell is in a state of repose when it rejects sodium and accepts potassium. It is in an active state when accepting sodium. This activity affects the nerves and causes insomnia. He described his success on treating sleeplessness by limiting or eliminating salt.

More evidence against the use of added salt is not hard to come by, but the above should convince anyone that salt is not conducive to good health. If your heart and kidneys are in good shape, stop using salt and help them stay that way. If you're already having such trouble, a salt reduction should improve your condition.

CHAPTER XLVIII

Is Mustard the Secret Killer?

A striking possibility has been raised that important types of heart disease could be associated with the regular eating of large amounts of table mustard.

Does the thought surprise and shock you? It does us too, in spite of the fact that for years now *Prevention* has been pointing out the dangers of strong spices and warning readers against them. Yet it never occurred to us, as it has hardly occurred to anyone, that a simple spice could cause anything so serious as a deadly heart attack. Nor is it yet proven that it will. But a very good case for an association has been made out by a Cleveland doctor, Jackson Blair, M.D., of the medical staffs of Lutheran and St. John's Hospitals in Cleveland. Writing in the *Ohio State Medical Journal* (August, 1965) Dr. Blair describes in full the personal observations that have led him to believe mustard is the hidden killer for which medical science has been searching.

Dr. Blair's paper lists 12 cases of heart attack that he

has personally attended, in all of which the patients were found to be unusually large eaters of mustard:

Case Histories

1. M. K., a man of 49 now, had a coronary thrombosis (damaging passage of a blood clot through the heart) at the age of 45. He had eaten at least one sandwich with mustard on it a day for about 20 years and also used mustard on his eggs, which he ate daily.

2. J. A. S., a man of 55, used mustard on sandwiches every day and also ate it frequently with ham and sausage, as well as eating considerable mayonnaise containing mustard. He had a heart attack.

3. W. A., a man of 36, used to mix powdered mustard with beer to make it taste stronger and ate large quantities of mustard on hot dogs, ham sandwiches and hamburgers, which he consumed often. He had a coronary attack at 34.

4. J. L. B., a man of 45, had sandwich lunches with mustard on them 90 per cent of the time. He had acute coronary thrombosis and infarction (hemorrhage in the heart caused by a blood clot).

5. H. G., a woman of 49, had eaten a sandwich with mustard on it every day for nine years and also ate a lot of hot dogs and hamburgers with mustard. She had an acute coronary attack and infarction.

6. W. B., a man, loved cheese and ham and ate them often with a great deal of mustard. He also used a great deal of mayonnaise. He had an acute coronary thrombosis at the age of 41.

7. F.J., a woman, frequently ate hog dogs with mustard and used mayonnaise at least twice a week on salad

[399]

greens and on potato salad. She died at the age of 59 of acute coronary thrombosis and infarction.

8. L. K., a man who ate two or three hot dogs every night with mustard, used a lot of pepper on his food, and drank a lot of ginger ale, had acute coronary thrombosis and infarction at the age of 48.

9. W. L., a man who ate two hamburgers every day, covered with mustard, for two years, had acute coronary thrombosis with infarction at the age of 49.

10. E. D., a man who liked to eat cold meats with large amounts of mustard for lunch and often for evening snacks, suffered two heart attacks and died of the second.

11. F. D., a man who was very fond of ham and ate it at least once or twice a week for many years, always with mustard, survived his first heart attack but had a second and died.

12. A man whose favorite pastime was to sit in front of his TV with a bag of pretzels and a jar of mustard, eating pretzels and mustard all evening, died of coronary thrombosis with infarction at the age of 50.

Dr. Blair states that "It is the author's opinion that mustard is the dietary agent responsible for the primary injury leading to the coronary atherosclerosis and probably responsible in some cases to triggering the thrombosis."

Reviewing his evidence, he points to an earlier study he made showing 50 cases of high blood pressure in excessive users of pepper, mustard and ginger. This was later confirmed by a laboratory study in which it was shown that high blood pressure could be produced in rats with these spices.

[400]

Of the three, Dr. Blair reports that mustard contains the highest proportion of a poisonous volatile oil which he considers the responsible agent. He goes on to state that oil of mustard has a strongly injurious effect upon the walls of the capillaries and can cause ulceration of the skin.

He believes it can also cause ulceration inside an artery, in this way inducing the formation of a blood clot which travels to the heart and causes an attack. Dr. Blair also points out that the United States, which leads the world in its incidence of heart attacks, is an enormous consumer of mustard having used 53 million pounds of mustard seed in 1960, a figure that has undoubtedly grown since then. He also points out that wherever there has been a reduced incidence of heart disease accompanying a reduced consumption of fats or sugars, there has simultaneously been a reduced consumption of mustard.

Dr. Blair's paper is not a conclusive scientific demonstration. It involves no control studies nor does it involve large numbers of people. Nevertheless, the personal observations of talented doctors made in just this way have often resulted in significant advances in medical knowledge. It was in this way that the use of digitalis in heart disease and vaccination for smallpox were first discovered. Penicillin emerged from the same kind of personal observation and there is a distinct possibility that Dr. Blair's observation on the relationship between the eating of strong spices, particularly mustard, and heart disease will also take its place as a significant discovery that will help us all to have stronger and healthier hearts.

[401]

CHAPTER XLIX

Fluoridation and Your Heart

We cannot claim to be sure of the fact, but there is a persistent rumor that since fluoridation was begun in Newburgh, New York, some 17 years ago, the rate of heart disease deaths in that city has become the highest in New York state. We do not like to report unconfirmed rumors ordinarily. We have been trying for two years to get figures on Newburgh that would give us some official tally on the incidence of disease and causes of death. There has been such a complete lack of cooperation on every official level that we have indeed come to think that the facts are being deliberately concealed from the public.

Grand Rapids, Michigan, has been drinking fluoridated water since 1946. According to the latest figures of the Michigan Department of Health, which are for the year 1962, in that year Grand Rapids had 814 deaths because of heart disease. Nearby Flint, a city

[402]

that has never had fluoridated water, and is slightly larger than Grand Rapids, had only 664 deaths from the same cause in the same year. Grand Rapids, with nearly 20,000 fewer people according to the 1960 census, had nearly 23 per cent more deaths from heart disease.

Now such a comparison, of course, does not necessarily prove anything. The greater incidence of deaths from heart disease in Grand Rapids might quite possibly be no more than coincidence so far as fluoridation is concerned. A scientific study of the reason, for example, might find out that the people of Grand Rapids smoke more cigarettes or that the air of that city is more polluted. It might. On the other hand, it just might find out that fluoridated water really is the cause that more people in Grand Rapids are dying of heart disease.

A statistical comparison such as we have just made does not prove anything, but it does point out strongly the need for investigation and study to determine scientifically whether fluoridated water causes heart disease or is as harmless as its proponents claim. Has such a study ever been made? Not to our knowledge. We have received many bland assurances that are no more than opinions without scientific backing. The facts are either unknown or being kept remarkably quiet.

However, we have just received rather frightening confirmation of the suspicion we have long held that fluoridated water may be causing some of the increase in heart disease that is plaguing the United States. This

[403]

confirmation comes from an unimpeachable source. It is a symposium of top notch scientists that was conducted in Bern, Switzerland, October 15 to 17, 1962. Recently published by Schwabe and Company, Basel, Switzerland, under the title "The Toxicology of Fluorine," the study is a remarkably thorough and completely scientific exchange of information by experts in this field from all over the world. It is not an easy one to read. The articles it contains are in German, French and Italian in addition to those in English. But it is well worth the reading for anybody who really wants to know the scientific facts about fluorine.

It was among the papers of this symposium that we found one highly illuminating study of the effect of fluorine on the heart by a Japanese scientist, T. Takamori, of Gifu Medical College, Gifu, Japan.

It should be understood that this symposium was not concerned with the question of fluoridation as such. As explained in the editor's preface, by Professor T. Gordonoff, M.D., of the University of Bern, although fluorine is known to be one of the most toxic elements on earth, very little is actually known about the mechanisms of its toxicity and the precise levels involved. And it was to study this deep scientific problem, rather than the political problem of fluoridation, that the symposium was organized. "We invited representatives of all those sciences concerned with toxicological research of fluorine who had opportunity to collect personal data during the research on this element. Present were chemists, agricultural chemists, botanists,

[404]

veterinarians, pharmacists, pathologists and clinical physicians."

Professor Takamori who discussed his studies of the effects of fluorine on the heart is an M.D.

His paper begins by pointing out that there has been hardly any investigation of this question. The only studies he was able to cite are two by other Japanese investigators, made in 1952 and in 1954. One of these, the 1954 study by Okushi, had found that among inhabitants of high fluorine districts there was both electrocardiographic and x-ray evidence of heart damage, consisting of swelling of the heart tissue and enlargement of that organ.

Of course, if you want to study the effect of fluorine on the heart, it is not possible to take human subjects and feed them this poison to see what happens to them. The accepted scientific procedure is to conduct thorough studies on laboratory animals whose metabolic reactions with regard to the particular experiment are known to be strongly similar or identical to those of man. Professor Takamori used rats and rabbits.

Another standard technique is to give the laboratory animal a higher dosage for a shorter period of time, this being very carefully computed to give a result in about two months that would be equivalent to what happens to man under the circumstances being tested over a period of many years.

"The observed heart changes were marked regressive degeneration of myocardial fibres such as cloudy swelling and vacuolar degeneration, infiltration of round cells in interstitial tissue and small hemorrhages in

[405]

several places. The degree of the changes was correspondingly proportionate to the length of administration and dosage of sodium fluoride." The changes at a dosage equivalent in effect to what happens to human beings drinking fluoridated water over a period of years were comparatively mild. But there were definite changes, showing as a cloudy swelling of the heart on x-rays and as weakening of the cell structure. In rabbits there was also a thickening of the inner walls of the heart, abnormal retention of water in the heart tissue and numerous small hemorrhages.

This is not to say that fluoridation of municipal water at a level of one part per million is going to give everybody heart disease. If that were the case, everybody in Grand Rapids and Newburgh might already be dead. But it does seem to be giving heart disease to an increased number of people after 15 years of fluoridation. How many more will suffer weakening of their hearts after 20 years of drinking fluoridated water? And how many after 30 years?

We do not know the answer. But we certainly feel it is high time that our Public Health Service at least began to study this question. It is time some responsible authority made a beginning toward finding the answer.

Part Nine:
STRESS

CHAPTER L

Emotional Strain and the Heart

It is typical of our society that we insist on simple answers to complicated questions. This is especially so in questions of health. When people ask what causes cancer, they don't want to be told that it is a combination of things, such as ingested poisons, food that is denatured, missing nutrients, etc. They want a pat answer—one thing: smoking, liquor, polluted air or fried foods. They want to be assured that if they avoid any one of these, cancer will pass them by. The attitude is similar for all of our major diseases.

In the field of heart disease research, the answers seem to be more confusing than in any other, because the emotions are involved as well as diet, exercise and other factors. An article in the *Journal of the American Medical Association* (October 3, 1959) describes one of the scientific studies which showed emotional strain to be a force involved in the onset of heart disease.

[409]

It is not the only cause, and may not be a cause at all in some individuals, but observations indicated to Dr. Henry I. Russek, M.D., that one who suffers from emotional strain is more likely to suffer from coronary disease than one who does not. As a matter of fact, Dr. Russek's findings put emotional stress above diet, smoking, heredity, obesity and lack of exercise as a cause of heart trouble.

How Dr. Russek arrived at this conclusion is interesting. In association with a colleague, he carefully assessed the background of 100 heart patients under 40 years of age. In 91 per cent of them prolonged emotional strain associated with job responsibility preceded the attack. In a group of 100 patients suffering from diseases other than heart disability, and used as controls for comparison, only 20 per cent were found to be under similar strain preceding the serious attack of their particular illness.

Further study of Dr. Russek's findings leads one to believe that a heart disease victim follows a definite pattern of personality. For example, 46 per cent of the 100 heart patients worked sixty or more hours per week; aside from this group, another 25 per cent were holding two jobs at the time of the attack. In another 20 per cent there was unusual fear, insecurity, discontent, frustration, restlessness, or a feeling of inadequacy in relation to employment.

Further comparison between the heart patients and controls revealed that the heart cases more frequently held positions of responsibility or jobs involving pressure due to deadlines than did the controls. How-

[410]

ever, in some cases cause of stress was laid not to the type of work, but to too many hours of work a week, or to secondary stresses in so-called leisure time.

The theory of work-approach-heart-disease relationship was studied from a different angle by Friedman and Rosenman. They compared groups of men selected solely according to behavior pattern routinely shown at work. Group I showed intense striving, an inclination to compete, desire for recognition, unusual mental and physical alertness, and involvement in deadlines. Group II had a behavior pattern opposite to I. Group III was similar to Group II, but complicated by a chronic state of anxiety or insecurity.

Friedman and Rosenman found coronary disease seven times more frequent in Group I (the anxious ones) than in Groups II and III. It is noteworthy that 80 per cent of this group showed obvious characteristics that were easily connected with mental attitudes, such as rapid body movement, tense facial musculature, explosive conversational intonations, hand or teeth clenching, excessive unconscious gesturing and a general air of impatience.

Dr. Russek's findings were contrary in the latter respect. While some of the 100 patients showed some or all of these characteristics, most had a striking degree of self-control, dignified reserve and complacency.

Essentially, over-conscientiousness and taking their work too seriously were the marks of Dr. Russek's 100 heart patients. Either a desire for recognition or a deep sense of obligation to employer or family could be found in most of them. They were generally too

[411]

concerned about time, overmeticulous, concerned about trivia, impatient with subordinates, worrisome, unwilling to delegate authority. Responsibilities on domestic, occupational and social levels were assumed by these people beyond the dictates of good judgment, and they were prone to neglect the prudent rules of good health.

Is diet not involved at all? Dr. Russek says it is a factor. He advocates a low fat diet, especially for one involved in a stressful situation, either occupationally, domestically or socially. By way of illustration he points to Norway and the Netherlands during World War II. It was a most stressful time for the people of these countries, yet there was no increase in the death rate due to cardiac disease. Dr. Russek regards the fact that fat foods were not generally available to the people at that time, as a partial explanation. In America today the cardiac death rate goes up steadily and it could be due to stress complicated by the fact that many Americans indulge in the readily available high fat diet.

That factors other than stress can influence the onset of heart disease is not disputed. Of the 100 heart patients observed by Dr. Russek, every one had high fat diet, heredity factor, or emotional strain in his background. Of the controls, 24 per cent were entirely free of any of these. The heart patients were found to have two of these major factors in the background of 95 per cent of the 100 cases. Of the controls, only 12 per cent had two such factors.

Dr. Russek checked on smoking and found that not only was smoking more prevalent in the coronary group, but twice as many of the coronary patients, as

[412]

compared with the controls, were heavily addicted to the use of tobacco. It was undecided by the author whether the smoking brought on the heart disease, or whether it was a manifestation of the inner tensions usually present in a coronary-prone subject. Nervous smoking, as well as eating and drinking, may be the result of stressful situations. Social activities can often breed the feeling that only a cigarette, a drink or food will fill the anxious or boring moment. If one is continually thrown into such situations, the habit is easily formed which eventually affects one's health and perhaps one's heart.

If Dr. Russek's deductions on the basis of observing 100 cardiac patients are not scientifically absolute, they certainly are indicative of stress as a factor in heart disease. He even quotes authorities to show that the cholesterol level of the blood rises strikingly during stressful situations. Emotional episodes call forth rapid mobilization of fatty acids from body tissues into the blood stream. Stress is related in this, and other known and unknown ways, to changes in the body's workings. It is not difficult then to attribute heart disease to a steady disruption of normal body functions by constant and unrelieved stress.

We have often emphasized the connection between the emotions and diet. The B vitamins have been shown time and again to have an almost miraculous control over healthy mental attitudes. If tenseness and emotionalism seem to be creeping into your make-up, if you find yourself slipping into the personality pattern described above, check into your diet. Do you include brewer's yeast, desiccated liver, wheat germ and the organ meats, all rich in B vitamins? Do you find yourself eating more and more refined foods, starches, bread and sweets which are devoid of these precious nutrients or rob the few you've managed to acquire? Are you hurrying through breakfasts of coffee and sweet rolls, and lunches of sodas, sandwiches with jelly or processed cold cuts, and a candy bar? Is dinner a starchy frozen meat pie or spaghetti topped off with pie and ice cream? This kind of eating does not prepare one to deal calmly with the stresses of family and job. This kind of eating can lead to heart disease.

CHAPTER LI

The Pace of Modern Living

J. I. Rodale

Mike Labanc died of a heart attack in his sleep some time ago. He was not a very old man and his friends were amazed when they heard of his death. Mike was night watchman at my electrical factory at Emmaus, Pennsylvania, and was one of the most easy-going of men you would ever want to meet. He was a person who was burdened with few of the character-istic mental tensions that people generally believe are killing us. I recall his coming into my office on several occasions to show me some beautiful specimens of vege-tables that grew in his organic garden. I can still see his friendly, gentle smile as he expounded on his gardening methods.

No sir! Mike was not one who was beset with any

stresses and strains; so why did he die of a heart attack at such an unripe age?

This set me to wondering and doing a little observing of this so-called fast-moving age of ours, and I was astounded at the lack of pace that I found when I began to look for it.

Here was a man who lived in a peaceful rural community, who went through life at a reasonable pace, who spent pleasant hours in his vegetable garden, but who died from a disease that is supposed to be attributed to the nerve-racking tensions of our worry-killing age. The more I thought of it the more I became convinced that it was something else that killed Mike Labanc, not a fast pace.

When one talks about the alarming increase of heart disease deaths, whether it be to a physician or to a layman, one invariably gets the same opinion: it is due to the fast pace at which we are living. You will get this answer 100 times out of 100. But it is a glib statement, given with a positive assurance, and not based on firsthand knowledge of the facts upon which an opinion can be based. The person has not predicated his view on a thorough understanding of what went on in previous times, as compared to today.

Even old folks, who should know better, fall in with the common fallacy, that conditions today are more tense than they ever were. But their memories are dulled by the cobwebs of age, like the old lady at Dingley Dell who said to Mr. Pickwick, "Ah, Mr. Pickwick, young people was very different when I was a girl." But actually, were they? As Arthur J. Snider

[416]

points out in his column in the *Chicago Daily News*
(Nov. 26, 1955: "The people of one age are little
different than those of another. Each age has its own
stresses. While not the same for each age, they are a
constant factor."

A magazine of a previous era, called *The Horseless
Age,* referred to the "tired nerves of this overwrought
generation." This is a period which we describe as a
peaceful horse-and-buggy era. Yet the nerves of the
people of that time were considered overwrought by the
imagined stresses and strains of those days. There hasn't
been a generation in this giddy, fantastic world of ours
that didn't consider itself more overwrought than the
people who came before it.

Can you picture Noah when the flood came? When
God told him he was going to drown everyone but his
family? That was sufficient to imprint that generation
with the word *overwrought* in big capital letters. And
can you see the reaction of Moses when he came down
from Mt. Sinai, seeing his own brother shattering a
lifetime of work and ideals, in the midst of an idol-
worshipping ceremony? Can you imagine King David
who inherited the primitively crude organization of
King Saul, faced with a disunited Israel, with enemies
from within and without his country ready to attack
him? He must have said that Saul had a bed of roses
compared to his tribulations. Or Julius Caesar, or
George Washington or Abraham Lincoln. Each one
of these men no doubt was of the opinion that his
predecessors had it much easier.

Listen to Thomas Love Peacock, an English novelist

[417]

of a hundred years ago, ridiculing the "hectic" speed of his generation: "Thirty-nine years ago steamboats were just coming into action and the railway loco-motive was not even thought of. Now everybody goes everywhere, going for the sake of going, and rejoicing in the rapidity with which they accomplish nothing."

Hidden in the interior of his diatribe is an admission that his age was faster, and therefore somewhat more nerve-racking than those which went before. Human character has not changed. We of this generation think ourselves more overwrought than the people of previous generations. It is given to us in newspapers, from the pulpit, the rostrum, the school, and in dozens of other places, so that when Uncle Gus suddenly keels over from a heart attack, and the doctor sagely advises that he died from the heavy strain of the modern pace, we don't doubt him for a moment.

Man has been a creature of fallacy ever since time began. It seems inherent and almost instinctive in his make-up to believe in false things. Straight, unvar-nished facts seem to be too dull for his appetite. Better an interesting fallacy than a stupid truth. There is overwhelming evidence that man likes to be hoaxed.

In the field of medicine especially, man seems to delight in being completely taken in by the numerous, venerable and deep-rooted but erroneous beliefs that are clung to with an unshakable determination, because they are vouched for by the authorities. But every generation of doctors discredits dozens of medical axioms, beliefs and procedures of previous medical generations.

[418]

When we hear of a prominent business executive dying of a heart attack at an early age we immediately ascribe it to the high pressure of our times. And when large numbers of executives of big corporations such as Du Pont and General Motors drop dead of heart disease, it is easy to jump to a conclusion about it. We picture these executives as engaged in an incessant battle of business. We consider them under terrific strains. Therefore, *ipso facto,* the strain is killing them. *Fortune* magazine (June, 1950) published an article entitled "Why Executives Drop Dead," which considers the tensions and pressures of their work as the underlying cause of their early deaths. But nothing can be further from the truth.

In the *Wall Street Journal* of May 9, 1957, there is an article headed, "Bosses Ail No More Than Other Employees, Company Medic Says." The article goes on, "In a just-released survey of industrial physicians most of the doctors reported 'no evidence' that executives are in any worse state of health than other employees. In fact, noted Dr. C. A. D'Alonzo, assistant medical director of E. I. Du Pont de Nemours & Company, Du Pont's top men seem less likely than other employees to suffer from heart disease and high blood pressure."

In the same survey, and speaking about Health Research Center in Chicago, Dr. Charles Thompson, head of the center, said that heart disease is more closely associated with executives than with lower-rung employees because "once an executive has it, he's a marked man. He gets his name in the papers and everybody knows about it. But a plumber could die of coronary disease and nobody would know about it but his family and his union."

One doctor in the survey noted that it is true that executives must decide big problems. "But," said he, "it's no harder for a vice president to decide on a $20,000 deal than for a foreman to decide on a $20 deal. In fact, the $20 may be more real to the foreman."

Further in this survey an organization called The Life Extension Examiners stated that "executives were in pretty good shape physically and that all the talk about their health troubles was damaging them emotionally." So we see that we have work to do in dispelling the fallacy that this pace is killing us.

Another argument against the conception that pace kills is the fact mentioned by Dr. Paul D. White, heart consultant to former President Eisenhower, that the danger of heart disease is no greater for big-city dwellers than for country folk. Speaking jointly with Dr. A. Wilbur Duryee, president of the New York Heart Association, he said, "There is no evidence that heart disease is more prevalent in the metropolitan area, with which tensions are associated, than in the country at large."

Another bit of evidence: In Chicago the heart death rate per hundred thousand of white persons aged from 46 to 64 years was 71. For Negroes the comparative figure was 831. This is quoted in the November 21, 1955 issue of *Medical News,* and Dr. Walter C. Alvarez, commenting on it said, "This certainly does not support the idea that the commonest cause of heart attacks is the strain of life in big business."

[420]

Yet, in reading medical journals and other publications, I continually see references to the stresses and strains of our lives as a factor predisposing to heart disease. A typical one is in *The New York Times* (Oct. 28, 1957) which said that, "At the American Heart Association's annual Scientific session, evidence was presented from human tests that stresses imposed by modern business competition were responsible for blood patterns predisposing to heart ailments."

The Medical Press (London), November 20, 1957, in an editorial states, "Never before in the history of this country has mental stress and strain been so great." Shades of Oliver Cromwell!

People usually see vividly only what is directly under their noses. The past is a romantic blur seasoned with glamorized misconceptions based on the popular literature and the hearsay of careless tongues. So, we build up a common belief that we are all traveling at a high speed, harassed with mental tensions which cause heart disease, ulcers, and increased pulses. We have built up a notion that compared to us, our predecessors of the eighties were crawling snails. We look back nostalgically on the last generation as living in a heavenly Garden of Eden, a blissful sort of horse-and-buggy existence which was like a golden dream, when no one worried about anything and people sat around cracker barrels twiddling their thumbs idly, and having a generally enjoyable time of it.

According to this picture, today we are working our knuckles off on life's hectic battlefront where people are being knocked off with heart disease right and left

[421]

because of the rigors of the fast pace under which they are living. Well, if this is the picture *you* have in your mind's eye, then you are due for a rude awakening. But perhaps I should not have used the word rude, because when your spirit becomes disabused of this absurd illusion, a tremendous load will come off it. You will become a freer person, relieved of the tormenting fear that your pace is slowly killing you. Such a fear can do no good.

CHAPTER LII

Stressful Episodes

J. I. Rodale

The fact that stresses that arise in our daily lives can be a factor inimical to good heart health came forcefully home to me one day at the Hialeah race track at Miami, Florida. Some friends had dragged me there and under conditions of propinquity I put $25 on a horse. He was a 10 to 1 shot, and as I saw him edging ahead, and realized that I might win $250, I began to experience some terrific angina pains. It wasn't the money, it was the excitement of winning. My horse *did* win by a good margin, but it was a rather close call for me. Had it not been that I am a regular taker of heavy doses of vitamin E, along with eating what I consider the proper diet for a heart case, and walking an hour a day, I believe my number would have been up that day. So, today, when I read that

[423]

stresses and strains are a factor in heart disease, I pay attention.

Let us see what some physicians think on this subject. Dr. Herman T. Blumenthal, laboratory director of St. Louis Jewish Hospital, as reported in *Newsweek* for April 16, 1956, believes that emotional stress is the main cause of arteriosclerosis, or hardening of the arteries. For what reason? He claims that stress raises the blood pressure. It is not normal high blood pressure that damages the artery walls, but the characteristic fluctuations in it, caused by stress and strain—the ups and downs. Fluctuations of blood pressure against artery walls cause injuries and hardening. To be healthy, artery walls should be elastic. A significant remark made by Dr. Blumenthal: "Except for a small number of persons who have inherited abnormal amounts of fat in their bloodstream, cholesterol is the result, not the cause of the disease."

Dr. Hans Selye in his famous book *Stress* (Acta, Inc.) states that emotional excitement leads to the increase of the pulse rate and blood pressure and causes a shrinking of the arteries. Fear will markedly reduce the flow of blood in the body. In experiments, says Dr. Selye, repeated emotional stimuli caused an inflammation of the external sheath of arteries which is the reason why various stresses cause angina pains. "Many other experimental and clinical observations suggest that nervous strain can cause arteriosclerotic lesions."

Situations provocative of frustration and anger raise the blood pressure, says Dr. Selye, and reduce the blood flow to and from the kidneys. Studying 695 men of an armored brigade which took part in desert warfare for one year, it was found that 27 per cent had high blood pressure at rest for months after this period.

Dr. George Calver, attending physician to congressmen and senators in Washington, said, as reported in *Parade* of April 15, 1956: "Heart attacks are brought on by what is technically known as the 'serum cholesterol'—blood solids that clog arteries. Tensions and strains that produce high blood pressure should be avoided, because serum cholesterol is 5 times greater when the blood pressure is high than under normal pressure."

The *Parade* article then describes how Representative Michael Edelstein (D) of New York died in the lobby of the House of Representatives five minutes after a bitterly controversial exchange with Congressman John Rankin (D) of Mississippi.

Dr. Calver states: "Emotional stress can produce a change in the hormone pattern, a change in the gland secretions. They may be increased or decreased, or there may be a stoppage. There are cases in which the entire intestinal tract has been paralyzed by anger. These changes in gland secretions may cause heart spasms which are fatal."

But take my own case at the race track. Had I not been taking massive doses of vitamin E, would they have carried me out of the place that day? My suggestion is that all congressmen, all statesmen, all public officials be furnished vitamin E by the Government. It will save money in the long run.

Dr. Calver offers some excellent advice as a general

[425]

means of helping the heart. "You have to walk enough to burn up the excess energy produced by food," he advises. "The man who eats and exercises regularly has a 100 per cent better chance than the other fellow to ward off heart trouble."

I have found that out also from personal experience. I walk an hour a day. But the effect of exercise on the heart is covered in another chapter.

According to Alan R. Moritz, M.D., writing in *The Journal of the American Medical Association* of December 4, 1954, the work of the heart is increased where there is emotional excitement. This is shown by an increase of the pulse and the systolic blood pressure. He says that in a normal heart there will be no trouble, but where the coronary arteries are narrowed through arteriosclerosis or other disease, there may be heart failure in a case of serious emotional disturbance. The increased work-load creates an oxygen requirement that cannot be furnished by the narrow arteries. The heart attack usually occurs soon after the emotional episode.

In the *Journal of the American Medical Association* of June 12, 1954, Smith and Chapman write of a simulated heart disease caused by anxiety. In other words, some persons are talking themselves into having symptoms of heart disease. According to one authority, 90 per cent of the soldiers in British army cardiac (heart) hospitals during World War I had no organic heart disease. The patient's fears and anxieties cause him to think he has heart disease—any minor discomfort is interpreted as a sign of disease. Such persons actually

[426]

develop palpitations, chest pain, and difficulty in breathing.

According to these authors, the best treatment for such cases is in some way to relieve their anxiety, to decrease their tensions. In my opinion if vitamin E were prescribed it would be far better, especially if it were accompanied by a thorough description of what it could do for the patient. That would be an effective way to subdue his fears and decrease his tensions. Perhaps the fact that these people worry easily may be due to the fact that they have many vitamin and mineral deficiencies, and the prescribing and use of a whole set of vitamins and minerals will give them a sense of physical well-being that would preclude the harboring of such imaginary anxieties.

The doctor can talk all he wants to, in order to attempt to relieve such people of their anxieties, but the effect will be only temporary. If there are deep-seated causes such as vitamin deficiencies, the symptoms will recur. If the doctor will apply the methods of this book, i.e., check on the patient's diet, reduce the carbohydrate content, stop him from smoking and using coffee, reduce his pulse by the methods we suggested, prescribe daily walks, and make him take calcium (bone meal), vitamins B, C, and E, he will give the patient a feeling that something is being done for him, and if he does all these things, something will really be accomplished.

Vitamins B and C especially are very important to counteract the effects of stress on the body. This subject is covered in the *Merck Reporter,* October, 1952, in an article by Drs. Goodhart and Jolliffe. According to this article, vitamin C is found in large amounts in the adrenal glands and is needed in additional amounts in adaptation to stresses. It states that the requirements for the B vitamins rise during stress.

If one has a heart condition or the symptoms just described, one must go into training so as to be able to cope with the occasional stresses that may arise. I follow and do all the things suggested in this book and feel certain that they will protect me under conditions of heavy mental and emotional strain.

I have mentioned the race track episode. There was another situation several years ago that almost was the death of me. I pride myself on being self-composed and well stabilized, but one day I made a scene at a meeting of directors in a corporation that I'm interested in, which was so violent, that if didn't have a heart attack then and there, it was a miracle of miracles. I do not wish to dwell on the details that led up to the scene. That was business, and sometimes people do things in business that they wouldn't do in a drawing room. I don't think I let myself go that way in 30 years. This was the most severe test of our system of nutrition, etc., that I could ever have undertaken. But it was the only way that I could accomplish the result I was after, and it succeeded and was for the good of the corporation involved.

I shall never forget it, my pulse and blood pressure must have shot skyhigh, and my breathing came with difficulty. Realizing the practical implications of my action—its effect on certain directors, I decided to

[428]

quit while I was ahead, and stomped out of the room followed by my son. When we got out into the hall I stopped and rested for a moment. I could feel my pulse going down and my breathing coming easier. In about two minutes I was as normal as any person could be, and let out a hearty laugh in celebration of what I had accomplished, for it was a good and honest purpose, which sometimes cannot be attained by legitimate means.

"Robert," I said, "were it not for my vitamin E and other vitamins and food supplements, you might have a dead man on your hands right now."

"I know it!" replied Robert.

Index

[431]

[432]

[433]